Retiree Health Benefits
Field Test of the FASB Proposal

Acknowledgments

The development of the Field Test methodology, the work done for each of the participating companies, and the compilation, summary, and analysis of the Field Test results required the efforts of numerous people within Coopers & Lybrand. Without the assistance of these people, it would not have been possible to complete a project of the scope and magnitude of this Field Test. In this regard, we wish to particularly acknowledge the outstanding efforts of Teresa A. McKenna and Debra Rudin.

In addition, the following individuals' efforts are also gratefully acknowledged: Ngoc Bao, Ronald Barlow, Amy Bergner, Kathy Bird, Robert Bazzini, William Chau, Carol Dutchak, Dennis Daugherty, Grace DiLello, Bernie Erickson, Jack Forstadt, Kenneth Friedman, Loretta Gerardi, John Glynn, Lisa Gockley, John Gribble, Paul Grimaldi, Gordon Grubbs, Charles Harris, Martha Hein, Sandra Hunt, Stuart Katchen, Anita King, Andrew Lawlor, Bede Lee, John Leigh, Robert McCarthy, James McCready, James McDonald, Ann Marie Maccini, James Meehan, Gerald Millman, Tom Mitchell, Kim Monturiol, Theodore Nussbaum, Stephen Ohanian, Martin Pepper, Richard Poccia, Grace Riina, John Schubert, Martin Staehlin, Richard Todd Stockard, Jennifer Strand, Sheree Swanson, Steve Verando, Ken Wong, and Janice Zimmerman.

We would also like to thank the Field Test companies for their participation and cooperation in this project. Moreover, the research team appreciates the guidance provided by the members of the FERF Steering Committee and particularly the efforts of Roland L. Laing, Research Director of FERF. Finally, we express our appreciation to Diana Scott, Project Manager, and the Financial Accounting Standards Board (FASB) members for their interest in and support of the Field Test.

Special Acknowledgment

The researchers would like to mention in particular the valuable contribution made by Murray H. Goldstein at the beginning of this project. His untimely death made it impossible for him to see the Field Test to its conclusion, but his insight and knowledge are evident throughout the study.

Retiree Health Benefits
Field Test of the FASB Proposal

Harold Dankner
Barbara S. Bald
Murray S. Akresh
John M. Bertko
Jean M. Wodarczyk

Coopers & Lybrand

A Publication of
Financial Executives Research Foundation

Financial Executives Research Foundation
10 Madison Avenue, P.O. Box 1938
Morristown, New Jersey 07962-1938

Copyright 1989 by Financial Executives Research Foundation

All rights reserved. No part of this book may be reproduced in any form
or by any means without written permission from the publisher.

International Standard Book Number 0-910586-74-8
Library of Congress Catalog Card Number 89-84509
Printed in the United States of America
First Printing

Financial Executives Research Foundation is the research affiliate of Financial
Executives Institute. The basic purpose of the Foundation is to conduct research and
publish informative material in the field of business management, with particular
emphasis on the practices of financial management and its evolving role in the
management of business.

The views set forth in this publication are those of the authors and do not
necessarily represent those of the FERF Board as a whole, individual trustees,
or the members of the Project Advisory Committee or the
Financial Accounting Standards Board or its members.

About the Authors

Harold Dankner, CPA—Mr. Dankner is a Partner and National Director of Technical Services for the Actuarial, Benefits, and Compensation Group of Coopers & Lybrand. He has over 20 years of diversified experience in employee benefits and had overall responsibility for this Field Test project. Mr. Dankner also co-authored the 1983 field test report, *Accounting for Pensions: Results of Applying the FASB's Preliminary Views.*

Barbara S. Bald, ASA, EA—Ms. Bald is a pension actuary with over 15 years of diversified experience in employee benefits, and is a Director in Coopers & Lybrand's National Actuarial Unit. She is responsible for actuarial technical support and research, and led the development of the valuation software utilized in the Field Test as well as software used to analyze the impact of SFAS No. 87.

Murray S. Akresh, CPA—Mr. Akresh is a Manager in the National Accounting and SEC Directorate of Coopers & Lybrand where he is responsible for formulating firm policy and technical communications regarding pensions and other postretirement benefits. He co-authored the 1985 FERF study, *Non-Pension Benefits for Retired Employees: Study of Benefits and Accounting Practices.*

John M. Bertko, FSA—Mr. Bertko is a health actuary and a Partner in Coopers & Lybrand's Actuarial, Benefits, and Compensation Group and has expertise in both conventional fee-for-service group insurance and alternative delivery systems. He is currently the Chairman of the Subcommittee on retiree benefit plans of the American Academy of Actuaries.

Jean M. Wodarczyk, FSA—Ms. Wodarczyk is a Director in Coopers & Lybrand's Actuarial, Benefits, and Compensation Group and has extensive experience as an actuary in the group benefits area, with particular emphasis in the health care field.

Project Advisory Committee

Lonnie A. Arnett
Vice President and Controller
Bethlehem Steel Corporation

Michael J. Gulotta
President and Chief Actuary
Actuarial Sciences Associates, Inc.

B. Clare Harris (chairman)
Vice President and Controller
Monsanto Company

Frederick J. Hirt
Executive Director of Cost Accounting,
Financial Reporting, and Property
   Accounting
The Upjohn Company

William J. Ihlanfeldt
Assistant Controller
Shell Oil Company

Paul B. Lukens
Vice President of Accounting, Research, and
   Industry Affairs
CIGNA Corporation

A. Herbert Nehrling, Jr.
Assistant Treasurer
E. I. du Pont de Nemours & Company

FASB Liaison
Diana Scott
Project Manager
Financial Accounting Standards Board

Jennifer Strand
Technical Services Coordinator
Coopers & Lybrand

Nancy K. Farlow
Publications Manager
Financial Executives Research Foundation

Contents

1	Executive Summary	1
2	Overview of Retiree Health Benefits	9
3	The FASB Exposure Draft	19
4	The Field Test: The Companies, Their Plans, the Measurement Process, and Implementation Problems	45
5	The Health Care Cost Trend and Other Assumptions	65
6	Valuation Results	81
7	Accounting for Income Taxes	125
8	Effect on Income, Liabilities, and Net Worth	135
9	The Impact of Medicare Catastrophic Coverage	147
10	Strategies for Cost Management and Plan Design	163
11	Funding and Legislative Outlook	179
12	Profiles of the Field Test Companies	189

1
Executive Summary

Rising health care costs have now become a major concern for every employer that pays the health care bills for its employees and retirees. In February 1989, the Financial Accounting Standards Board (FASB or the Board) issued an Exposure Draft (ED) of a proposed Statement of Financial Accounting Standards (SFAS), *Employers' Accounting for Postretirement Benefits Other Than Pensions,* that would establish a new standard by requiring accrual accounting for retiree health and other postretirement benefits such as life insurance.

Recognizing the need to help the FASB and other interested parties, the Financial Executives Research Foundation (FERF) sponsored a field test study conducted by Coopers & Lybrand to assess the impact of accounting for retiree health benefits. The study was limited to retiree health benefits because the measurement of these benefits is generally more complex and raises many more data and implementation problems than other postretirement benefits. Using benefit and cost data from 25 participating companies, a team of health and pension actuaries, accountants, benefit consultants, and other professionals from Coopers & Lybrand analyzed the impact of the proposed new standard and the measurement and implementation problems that could affect accounting for retiree health benefits.

Overall Impact of Accrual Accounting

If the FASB adopts the approach proposed in the ED, the financial statements of companies sponsoring postretirement benefit plans could be significantly affected.

- ☐ *Higher expense.* Expense under accrual accounting would be higher than under pay-as-you-go accounting (see chapter 6). The difference will vary from company to company, depending on specific company demographics, the richness of plan benefits, and the assumptions used to determine expense. For most Field Test companies with a significant number of retirees (referred to as a "mature" company), expense for their company's retiree health care plans ranged from two and one-half to greater than seven times higher (under the ED) than under pay-as-you-go accounting. For "highly mature" companies with almost as many retirees as active employees, expense ranged from less than two to six times current pay-as-you-go costs. For "immature" companies with few retirees, pay-as-you-go costs are minimal and, therefore, the multiple of pay-as-you-go costs was much higher.

- ☐ *No tax deduction.* The higher expense under accrual accounting would not generally be deductible under current tax laws because current tax deductions are generally based on actual benefit payments (see chapter 11).

- ☐ *Limited book tax benefit.* Under SFAS No. 96, *Accounting for Income Taxes,* a portion of the higher expense under accrual accounting may fall right to the "bottom line"—with no offsetting tax benefit—directly reducing net income (see chapter 7).

- ☐ *Significant recorded liabilities and reduced net worth.* Higher expense would both drive up recorded liabilities and reduce net worth, affecting a company's debt-to-equity and other key ratios (see chapter 8). Consequently, some companies could fail to meet restrictive covenants in their debt agreements. In addition, some financial analysts may immediately deduct from net income or stockholders' equity the disclosed but unrecorded obligation at the date accrual accounting is adopted (the transition obligation) in evaluating a company's financial position.

Caution: The specific impact on a particular company's financial statements—either at the time of initial application or in later years—cannot be predicted without substantial analysis. Understanding the impact of these proposed changes on an individual company requires detailed information about its plan(s) and an analysis of many factors, particularly existing benefit coverage, demographics, current health care claims experience, and actuarial assumptions.

Current Practice

A majority of U.S. companies now provide nonpension postretirement benefits, of which retiree health care is generally the most significant in terms of cost (see chapter 2). When these benefits were first offered, the costs were relatively small. However, as health care costs escalated and the benefits and number of retirees covered under these programs expanded, employer costs increased dramatically. Increased longevity, reduced Medicare reimbursement, and earlier retirement also contributed to higher employer costs. Nationwide, unfunded retiree health obligations have been estimated to be over $200 billion, with some estimates greatly exceeding that amount.

Because only a few companies follow accrual accounting for retiree health benefits, obligations relating to these plans are not currently included in the balance sheet of most companies. Many employers that account for retiree health benefits on a "pay-as-you-go" basis have not measured or evaluated the obligations for their retiree health plans. Some do not even separate current health benefit expenditures for retirees from those for active employees.

Employees eligible for retiree health benefits are typically limited to those who retire from the company and can immediately receive pension benefits by completing certain age and service requirements. Early retirees are generally offered the same health care benefits as active employees. Almost all plans adjust health coverage at age 65 to reflect Medicare. Many plans also provide lifetime coverage for the retiree's spouse and limited coverage for other dependents. Moreover, many plans require participants to pay some portion of the cost.

The FASB Exposure Draft

The FASB would require companies to switch to accrual accounting for postretirement benefits other than pensions by 1992 and would require a "minimum" liability to be recorded on the balance sheet by 1997 (see chapter 3). Because the FASB believes that an employee earns these benefits in exchange for service rendered to the company, the accrual for postretirement benefits should, in their view, take place during an employee's working career, not at the time of retirement or after retirement. Thus, pay-as-you-go (cash basis) and terminal accrual (accrue at retirement) approaches would no longer be acceptable.

The FASB's stated objectives are to:

- □ have reported income reflect the cost of postretirement benefits over the period they are earned by employees;

- make the balance sheet more informative and more complete by including a measure of the obligation to provide postretirement benefits;
- make reported amounts more comparable and understandable by mandating a single method for measuring the obligation and cost; and
- enhance disclosure of the extent and effects of an employer's undertaking to provide postretirement benefits.

The Measurement Process

To analyze the potential impact of switching to accrual accounting under the ED, the following basic measurement steps were completed with respect to each company participating in the Field Test (see chapter 4):

- examined existing plan materials to understand the retiree health benefit program;
- analyzed claims and demographic data to identify average per capita (retiree) costs for a one-year period;
- estimated and discounted future benefit payments based on average per capita costs and actuarial assumptions selected by participating Field Test companies; and
- projected obligations and expense to show the impact of the ED, and the sensitivity to changes in assumptions and accounting approaches.

Alternative Assumptions and Accounting Methods

Retiree health obligations and expense levels under the proposed statement can vary significantly depending on the actuarial assumptions used to measure retiree health care plan benefits (see chapter 6).

The health care cost trend—or the rate at which health care costs are expected to rise in the future—and the discount rate used to determine present values are generally the two most powerful actuarial assumptions. The higher the cost trend, the higher the obligation and expense. The opposite is true for the discount rate.

Alternate Cost Trend Assumptions

Based on the specific requirements of the ED, companies selected their "best estimate" of future health care cost increases to measure obligations and expense. In addition to the "best estimate" assumption, "optimistic" and "pessimistic" cost trend assumptions were modeled—as well as a one percentage point decrease in the "best estimate" rate—in order to analyze the sensitivity to this assumption. For almost all Field Test companies, first year expense generally changed 5 to 20 percent from the "best estimate" using these optimistic and pessimistic assumptions, with a one percentage point decrease generally resulting in a 7 to 22 percent decrease in first year expense.

Some observers of the FASB project are concerned that the results under the ED would not be reliable due to the uncertainty of projecting health care costs for many years into the future. Some alternative approaches that have been suggested to mitigate the issue of reliability would reduce first year expense as compared to the ED (see chapter 6).

- Current cost levels could be viewed as a minimum estimate of future costs (e.g., a 0 percent cost trend assumption). In this view, obligations and expense under accrual accounting would not have to rely on projections that might be viewed as unreliable and speculative. If discount rates based on the guidance in the ED were not reduced concurrently, first year expense under this approach would generally be 50 to 70 percent lower.

- The minimum estimate of future costs could be based on an assumption of future general inflation (e.g., a 4½ percent cost trend assumption) mitigating some concerns regarding reliability, while still adding a measure of future cost increases. This approach would generally lower the first year expense by 30 to 50 percent (again, not reducing discount rates).

- The cost trend could be based on expected health care price inflation only (e.g., a 6 percent cost trend assumption rather than an all-encompassing health care cost trend of 8 percent) emphasizing that future cost increases due to changing technology and utilization patterns are difficult to project based on past experience. This approach would generally lower the first year expense by 15 to 30 percent (not reducing discount rates).

- Current cost levels could be used to approximate future costs (a 0 percent cost trend assumption), with a corresponding assumed discount rate of 0 percent. In effect, this approach is similar to the first alternative above, but with no discounting. This approach would either increase or decrease the transition obligation, depending on the direction and amount of spread between the assumed cost trend and discount rates under the ED. First year expense would generally be 30 to 50 percent lower than under the ED because interest cost would be eliminated under a nondiscounted approach.

Under all of these alternative approaches, the pattern of future years' expense will be significantly different than under the ED, depending on the approach selected to account for actuarial gains and losses. Because health care costs are expected to rise, large actuarial losses may arise in future years under these approaches.

Alternate Discount Rate

Some observers of the FASB project believe that the discount rate assumption should not be based on a hypothetical settlement of the obligation as called for under the ED. Generally, there are no settlement vehicles currently available for retiree health obligations that are similar to the annuities used to settle pension benefits. As a result, some believe that the discount rate should be based on a company's specific cost of borrowing or cost of capital since the "settlement" will use internal company funds generated by the business. Accordingly, each Field Test company was asked to select a company-specific discount rate. The company-specific rates selected were generally one to three percentage points higher than the ED rate. Using this rate reduced first year expense by 3 to 32 percent.

Alternate Attribution Period

The ED would require that companies use a single method to allocate the cost of a participant's benefits to individual years of service. Costs would generally be allocated from date-of-hire to the earliest date the employee is fully eligible for benefits (the attribution period). The FASB believes that this approach is appropriate since the employee does not "earn" any additional benefits based on service beyond the full eligibility date. Some observers of the FASB project have called for the attribution period to extend to the employee's expected date of retirement (the full-service period). Using a full-service attribution period was found to reduce first year expense by 1 to 21 percent, depending on specific company demographics, plan provisions, and retirement date assumptions.

Alternate Transition Approaches

Under the ED, the transition obligation would be amortized to expense on a straight-line basis over the average remaining service period of active employees (15 years may be used, if longer). Alternate approaches, not including immediate recognition, include the following:

Longer amortization period. Some observers are concerned that the proposed transition amortization period is too short to mitigate the effect of switching to accrual accounting and that a longer period, such as 30 years, may be appropriate. Lengthening the period over which the transition obligation is amortized to 30 years decreased first-year expense under the ED by 2 to 20 percent.

Mortgage amortization technique. Similar to a mortgage-type approach used for pension funding purposes, the transition obligation was amortized using an approach that amortizes an increasing amount of principal each year. Under this type of approach, first year expense was reduced by 13 to 38 percent.

"Grandfathering" transition approach. Similar to an approach sometimes followed when new laws are passed, costs could continue to be expensed under the pay-as-you-go method for retirees at transition. The provisions of the ED would then apply to benefits expected to be paid to future retirees. Coupling this approach with a full-service attribution period reduced first year expense by 7 to 42 percent.

Implementation Issues

A significant finding of the Field Test is that, in many cases, existing information about the retiree health plans, demographics, dependency status, and medical claims data (see chapter 4) was unavailable or of poor quality. Some companies that wanted to participate in the Field Test could not do so because they did not have even minimal information needed to perform a valuation of their retiree health benefit program.

Based on the Field Test experience, some companies will need to spend a good deal of time and effort obtaining needed plan and demographic data to perform a retiree health valuation. Moreover, they will have to work with their insurance carriers or third-party administrators to obtain reliable retiree claims experience on either a detailed or summary basis.

The detailed methodology developed for the Field Test was designed to identify data and implementation problems and to provide the companies with underlying information related to their costs. Of course, the measurement of retiree health benefits is in an evolutionary stage and work will still need to be done to find practical solutions to some of these issues. In the future, additional methods and procedures are likely to be developed and tested that may make the measurement process less difficult.

Recommended Corporate Actions

The issues involved in accounting for retiree health benefits are complex and should be addressed not only from a financial reporting viewpoint but also from a broader business perspective. Since virtually every employer sponsoring a retiree health benefit plan would be affected, companies should weigh the consequences of the FASB's proposal and consider taking positive steps to control health care costs and develop long-range solutions to human resource issues (see chapter 10).

The first step is to analyze the current costs of the company's health benefits program. A better understanding is needed regarding what the company is paying for today, the extent of health benefits, and the possible impact of the FASB's proposed accounting standard.

Then management can proceed to look for better ways to manage and control future costs while still providing competitive compensation and benefit packages. A thorough evaluation of health care cost reduction remedies—plan design changes, improved internal controls, and funding alternatives—should be performed, with the development of a detailed action plan.

Because of the current impact of increasing health care costs and the long-term policy implications involved, Coopers & Lybrand and the Financial Executives Research Foundation strongly urge companies to make their views known to the FASB through comment letters and oral presentations at public hearings. Companies may also wish to express their views to Congress and the administration regarding the related funding and tax issues.

2
Overview of Retiree Health Benefits

Twenty years ago, companies were mainly concerned with health care benefits for active employees. In the 1960s, Medicare assumed most of the costs of health benefits for retirees age 65 and over, so the costs to employers offering retiree health benefits were generally not significant. As benefits and early retirement incentives expanded, and more employees were given continued health care coverage after retirement, costs to employers increased dramatically. And, as costs rose, the share of benefits paid for by Medicare declined.

Magnitude of Unfunded Obligations

Today, retiree health benefits involve difficult business, social, and political issues, and have attracted increased attention. A primary reason for this increased interest is the significant size of estimated unfunded employer obligations. Until recently, most corporate executives did not know the extent of their company's retiree health benefit programs or the cash flows needed to finance these programs. Recent estimated projections for aggregate unfunded obligations for private employers to date have ranged from approximately $220 billion[1] to approximately $250 billion.[2] When future service is taken into account, the aggregate unfunded obligation is estimated at $402 billion.[3] Some estimates have greatly exceeded this amount. Of course, these and other estimates are very much dependent on the data and methodology used to produce the estimate; therefore, estimates must be viewed as general ranges.

As will be discussed in chapter 9, unfunded employer obligations may be decreased by expanded Medicare coverage of catastrophic illness. However, even with Medicare catastrophic coverage in effect, employer obligations will still be quite significant, estimated by the Employee Benefits Research Institute study to be at least $168 billion. That study also concluded that when public employers' obligations are added to estimated obligations for the private sector, the total estimated unfunded obligation to date (as adjusted for Medicare catastrophic coverage) is approximately $279 billion.[4]

Reasons for Increased Costs

These staggering estimates are but one piece of the complex issue of retiree health benefits. Recent economic and demographic trends have had—and may continue to have—a dramatic effect on the costs of retiree health plans. Since 1975, health care inflation has consistently outpaced general inflation, although there are year-to-year variations.[5]

Moreover, the population eligible for employer-provided retiree health benefits has grown significantly. The aging of the workforce, coupled with incentives for early retirement, have caused a large increase in the number of retirees covered by employer-sponsored health programs. Census projections for 1990 estimate that approximately 12.7 percent of the U.S. population will be over age 65.[6] By 2030, this percentage is expected to increase to over 21 percent[7] and further increases are anticipated as the "baby boom" generation matures. As a result, even greater numbers of individuals will be eligible for Medicare and employer-provided retiree health benefits, with perhaps fewer active workers to support them.

Costs for employer-provided retiree health benefits are also greater because increased life spans frequently result from the application of more advanced and more expensive medical technology. Retirees and their spouses are living longer, extending the period during which claims will be paid.

A related concern involves the gradual erosion of the Medicare program. Over the past several years, the share of health care costs for the elderly borne by Medicare has decreased, and Medicare has shifted primary payer responsibility to the individual and to other parties, such as employers, in many cases.

The Prevalence of Retiree Health Plans

In 1986, the U.S. Department of Labor found that approximately 76 percent of full-time employees of medium and large companies (those with at least 100 or 250 employees, depending on the industry) participated in health plans under which they could be eligible for retiree health benefits after retirement.[8] The 1985 FERF study found that 85 percent of large employers provided hospital and medical coverage to retired or terminated participants (see summary of survey results in table 2.1).[9]

For 1988, the U.S. General Accounting Office estimated that employer-sponsored retiree health plans covered about seven million retirees, at a cost to employers of about $9 billion.[10] However, retiree health benefits are not limited to employees of the largest U.S. companies—it is estimated that nearly half (42 percent) of the U.S. firms with 50 to 100 employees also provide some form of health benefits for retirees.[11]

TABLE 2.1 Survey of Prevalence of Employer-Sponsored Retiree Health Benefits

Benefits Provided to Retired or Terminated Participants	Prevalence	
	All Employers	Large Employers
Hospital/medical coverage	65%	85%
Dental benefits	18	19
Vision care benefits	Not Reported	4
Death benefits	50	71

The Nature of Retiree Health Benefits

Two groups of retirees are eligible to receive employer-provided health benefits: those age 65 and over and those under age 65 ("early retirees"). Early retirees are generally offered the same benefits as active employees. The Department of Labor found in 1986 that 78 percent of retirees under age 65 who received retiree health benefits had the same coverage as active employees, while 71 percent of retirees age 65 and over receiving health benefits had the same coverage as active employees (after considering the benefits provided by Medicare).

The costs for retirees age 65 and over and retirees under age 65 differ significantly because virtually all employer-sponsored plans are designed to coordinate or integrate with Medicare. Employer-provided health benefits for retirees age 65 and over are generally secondary to those provided by Medicare, and provide a supplement to Medicare coverage. Thus, the employer-provided portion is usually significantly reduced. In contrast, retirees under age 65 are generally not eligible for Medicare, and employer-sponsored health plans are the primary payers of health benefits for this group. Most plans require retirees to pay deductibles or coinsurance for their coverage, and some plans require retiree contributions for single or family coverage. Many plans provide spouses with lifetime coverage and may also cover other dependents. This family coverage feature can be very costly to the employer.

Eligibility for retiree health benefits varies from company to company, but it is frequently tied directly to eligibility for normal, early, or disability retirement under the company's pension plan. For example, when an individual is eligible to receive pension benefits (e.g., at early retirement after attaining age 55 and completing 10 years of service), the employee may also be eligible to receive retiree health benefits. While annual pension payments for early retirees are usually reduced because the payments must be spread out over a longer period than for those retiring at age 65, the employer's annual payments for retiree health benefits are not usually adjusted for early retirement. In fact, the early retirement causes additional postretirement benefit cost for the employer.

The FASB has likened retiree health benefits to pension benefits, concluding that retiree health benefits are a form of deferred compensation, as are pension benefits. Accordingly, the FASB concluded that accounting for these types of benefits should be similar. However, these two types of benefits also have many dissimilar characteristics. An employer's promise in a typical retiree health plan is made in terms of benefits or services to provide health coverage (e.g., hospitalization) to retirees regardless of cost. In contrast, an employer's promise in a typical pension plan is made in terms of dollars to provide a specified amount or level of benefits (e.g., 35 percent of final pay) to retirees. In a pension plan, an employer's commitment is either defined in terms of dollars or can easily be translated into dollars and quantified. However, in a retiree health plan, the actual cost of benefits generally will not be known until an illness occurs. In addition, costs can vary greatly by individual, and one individual may incur very different costs from one year to the next. The nature of the retiree health benefit thus makes measurement of the obligation much more difficult.

Table 2.2 compares some important features of pension and retiree health plans.

The Legal Environment

As individual companies confront the costs and financial reporting issues relating to their retiree health benefit programs, they may have legitimate business concerns about continuing their present programs. Some companies may decide to modify their benefits, or even cease providing retiree health benefits. Companies currently have considerable flexibility to change future benefits for active employees. However, as discussed more fully in chapter 10, the legal environment surrounding a company's ability to change or terminate benefits for current retirees is much more uncertain and complex. Conflicting court decisions indicate that, at a minimum, a company must have expressly reserved the right to modify or terminate these benefits in order to do so.

TABLE 2.2 Comparison of Pension and Retiree Health Benefit Plans

	Pension Plans	Retiree Health Benefit Plans	Comments
Measurement Characteristics			
Amount of plan benefits is definitely determinable.	Yes	No	Pensions are determined under a definite formula. Except for pension plans with automatic cost-of-living adjustments, the amount of a retiree's monthly benefit is fixed when payments commence. Generally, retiree health benefits are not precisely determinable until an illness or other event occurs. Duration of benefits are the same in pension and retiree health plans when both are payable during the lifetime of the retiree and/or spouse.
Records for benefit payments to retirees and beneficiaries are readily available.	Yes	No	For many companies, systems will need to be developed to maintain data on the health benefits paid to retirees and their dependents.
Plan Characteristics			
Specific eligibility criteria exist.	Yes	Yes	Age and service requirements are common.

TABLE 2.2 Comparison of Pension and Retiree Health Benefit Plans (continued)

	Pension Plans	Retiree Health Benefit Plans	Comments
Plan provides benefits that are earned ratably through employee's service period.	Yes	No	Retiree health benefit plans typically do not provide for benefit accruals or periodic vesting. Further, benefits generally are not tied to length of service.
Vesting of benefits required by statute.	Yes	No	Pension benefits accrue (earned by the participant) and vest in accordance with ERISA requirements. ERISA vesting requirements do not apply to retiree health benefits and case law is developing. No benefits are paid unless eligibility criteria are satisfied in typical retiree health plan.
Increases in real benefit cost after retirement are subject to close employer control.	Yes	No	For most retiree health plans, health care cost increases after retirement are heavily influenced by health care prices and other factors. Although the employer can control the health benefits covered under a plan, the utilization of specific coverages or procedures and the costs involved are generally beyond the employer's control. In addition, plans typically are coordinated with Medicare benefits and the employer has no control over future changes in the Medicare laws.

Other Characteristics

Plan termination is subject to regulatory controls.	Yes	No	Pension Benefit Guaranty Corporation does not regulate termination of retiree health plans.
Plan is subject to ERISA funding and benefit guarantee protections.	Yes	No	Companies filing for Chapter 11 Bankruptcy (reorganization) generally may not terminate current retiree health benefits.

TABLE 2.2 Comparison of Pension and Retiree Health Benefit Plans (continued)

	Pension Plans	Retiree Health Benefit Plans	Comments
Benefits typically are advance funded.	Yes	Not usually	Under ERISA, pension plans are required to be funded; however relatively few employers advance fund retiree health benefits.
Timing of accounting expense and tax deduction is generally consistent.	Not necessarily	Not necessarily	Unless funded, expense provisions for retiree health benefits generally would not be deductible until paid. Since pension plans are generally funded, expense and tax deductions are often consistent. However, under SFAS No. 87, pension expense and amounts funded are computed independently. For example, in some instances pension expense may have to be provided for financial reporting purposes even though tax-deductible plan contributions cannot be made if the employer has reached the full funding limitation under the Internal Revenue Code.
Obligation for accumulated benefits is generally considered in sale or acquisition negotiation.	Yes	Sometimes	Amount of obligation for retiree health benefits generally has not been available and sometimes had not been considered by acquirer in the past. These obligations are now being considered more frequently in acquisition deliberations.
Expense for plan is typically recognized on accrual basis.	Yes	No	See table 2.3 which illustrates current accounting practice.
Obligations are typically disclosed in financial statements.	Yes	No	Pension disclosures are required, but obligations for retiree health benefits have generally not been estimated.
Current and long-term obligations can be substantial.	Yes	Yes	

Current Accounting Practice

There are presently no specific requirements that all companies must follow in accounting for retiree health care plans. With few exceptions, retiree health care costs are currently accounted for as the claims are paid, on a pay-as-you-go basis (see summary survey results in table 2.3). For the most part, these obligations are not recorded on companies' balance sheets, although under current rules companies are required to disclose a description of the benefits, current accounting and funding policies, and the costs of benefits recognized for the period in their financial statements.

TABLE 2.3 Survey of Accounting Methods Used For Retiree Health Care Benefits by Large Companies[12]

	Cash Method[a]	Accrual Method	Terminal Accrual[b]	Not Disclosed[c]	Total Surveyed
Fortune 100 industrials	81	4	2	13	100
Retailing	11			13	24
Diversified services	3	2		5	10
Transportation	6	—	—	3	9
Total companies	101	6	2	34	143

a Referred to as the pay-as-you-go method
b Costs accrue at retirement
c Cannot determine whether nondisclosure is because there is no plan or because the costs of the plan are immaterial

Notes

1. U.S. General Accounting Office, "Future Security of Retirees' Health Benefits in Question," September 15, 1988, GAO/T-HRD-88-30.
2. Employee Benefit Research Institute (EBRI), "Issues and Trends in Retiree Health Insurance Benefits," November 1988.
3. U.S. General Accounting Office, "Future Security of Retirees' Health Benefits."
4. EBRI, "Issues and Trends."
5. U.S. Department of Labor, Bureau of Labor Statistics.
6. U.S. Department of Commerce, Bureau of the Census.
7. *Ibid.*
8. U.S. Department of Labor, Bureau of Labor Statistics, *Employee Benefits in Medium and Large Firms, 1986,* June 1987. See also, Michael A. Morrisey and Gail A. Jensen, "Employer Sponsored Post-Retirement Health Benefits: A Summary," University of Alabama at Birmingham, September 1988.
9. Coopers & Lybrand and Hewitt Associates, *Non-Pension Benefits for Retired Employees,* Financial Executives Research Foundation, 1985.
10. U.S. General Accounting Office, "Employee Benefits: Company Actions to Limit Retiree Health Costs," GAO/HRD-89-31BR.
11. Jonathan C. Dopkeen, "Postretirement Health Benefits," Health Services Research, 21:6, February 1987.
12. Coopers & Lybrand, *Retiree Medical Benefits: Understanding the Mounting Concern,* 1987.

3
The FASB Exposure Draft

On February 14, 1989, the FASB issued an Exposure Draft of a proposed Statement of Financial Accounting Standards entitled *Employers' Accounting for Postretirement Benefits Other Than Pensions*. The ED incorporates many of the concepts contained in SFAS No. 87, *Employers' Accounting for Pensions* and SFAS No. 88, *Employers' Accounting for Settlements and Curtailments of Defined Benefit Pension Plans and for Termination Benefits*. Currently, a codified and comprehensive set of rules detailing how employers should measure and account for nonpension postretirement benefits does not exist. Instead, employers rely upon prevalent practice in determining the generally accepted method of reflecting the cost of these benefits in financial statements.

This chapter provides an overview of the FASB and the standard-setting process and presents a brief history of the FASB project on postretirement benefits. It summarizes the significant accounting requirements contained in the ED and is designed to provide insight into the reasoning behind the FASB's proposal. Table 3.1 contains a comparison of the proposed accounting requirements in the ED to those of pension accounting under SFAS Nos. 87 and 88.

Introduction—The FASB

The FASB is the designated private sector organization responsible for establishing and improving standards of financial accounting and reporting. Organized in 1972, the FASB is independent of all other business, governmental, and professional organizations. Seven full-time members are appointed by the Board of Trustees of the Financial Accounting Foundation, the parent organization, and may serve up to two terms of five years each. The Foundation appoints FASB members from various professional backgrounds with the objective of achieving balanced viewpoints.

At the date of issuance of the ED, the FASB was comprised of two members from public accounting, two from industry, one from the federal government, one from education, and one who was a prior FASB director of research and technical activities (previously in public accounting).

The FASB determines the issues included in its agenda based upon the pervasiveness of the issue, the effectiveness of alternative solutions, technical feasibility of alternatives, and practical consequences. The FASB adheres to "due process" in setting accounting standards. First, a task force may be formed consisting of knowledgeable and interested people independent of the FASB who advise the FASB as necessary. Second, one or several discussion documents may be issued to inform and update the FASB constituency as to the issues, the scope of the project, other pertinent information and to solicit their views. This is often followed by public hearings to allow interested parties to testify directly to the FASB. The Board meets publicly to discuss and analyze the issues at hand. When a majority of the FASB members agree with the tentative conclusions on the issues, the FASB releases an exposure draft of the proposed standard and identifies a response period during which interested parties may submit written comments. Additional public hearings are often conducted subsequent to the comment period. The Board then publicly reconsiders its tentative conclusions based on those comments and testimony, and develops and votes on a final statement. A simple majority of the seven Board members is required to issue a statement of financial accounting standards.

Background and Scope

From 1979 to 1983, the FASB considered accounting for other postretirement benefits as a part of the pension accounting project. However, the Board decided in February 1984 that the accounting for these benefits should be evaluated separately and thus divided the project into pension and nonpension phases. The pension phase culminated with the issuance in December 1985 of SFAS Nos. 87 and 88 on employers' accounting for pensions.

In November 1984, the FASB issued SFAS No. 81, *Disclosure of Postretirement Health Care and Life Insurance Benefits*. This standard was issued as an interim measure in response to concerns over the lack of disclosures in employers' financial statements about those benefits. In April 1987, the FASB released Technical Bulletin (TB) No. 87-1, *Accounting for a Change in Method of Accounting for Certain Postretirement Benefits*. This TB is discussed in more detail later in this chapter.

The FASB believes that pension and postretirement benefits are similar in nature. The Board thus started with the presumption that postretirement benefits should be accounted for under the pension accounting rules in SFAS Nos. 87 and 88 unless it could be demonstrated that there are fundamental differences between other postretirement and pension benefits that would warrant different approaches. For the most part, the proposed measurement and transition requirements in the ED parallel those in pension accounting, except that the present value of expected postretirement benefits would be fully accrued by the date the employee is fully eligible to receive benefits (the eligibility date rather than at the expected retirement date).

The new standard would apply to employers providing postretirement benefits (such as health care, life insurance, or tuition reimbursement) to current and future retirees, their beneficiaries, and qualified dependents in accordance with the terms of a specified or implied funded or unfunded plan to provide such benefits. The ED also addresses settlement of the employer's postretirement benefit obligation and the curtailment of a benefit plan, as well as guidance in accounting for non-U.S. plans and business combinations. Other postemployment benefits, such as severance pay or wage continuation to disabled or terminated employees, are not covered by this proposed standard. The FASB may address the accounting for those benefits at some future date.

Though the requirements in the ED apply to a wide range of benefits offered to retirees, the remainder of this chapter and book will focus on the most complex of these benefits and the subject of the Field Test—retiree health benefits.

Accrual Accounting

Pay-as-you-go (cash basis) and terminal accrual (accrue at retirement) approaches would no longer be acceptable. The FASB believes that retiree health care, life insurance, and other postretirement benefits are forms of deferred compensation and, therefore, should be accrued while an employee works for the company. In the FASB's view, the accrual for the present value of future benefits should take place during an employee's working career up to the full eligibility date under the plan.

Eligibility Date Concept

The FASB approach to measurement is focused on three groups:

- retirees and dependents receiving health benefits;
- active employees fully eligible for retiree health benefits (for example, those eligible active employees beyond age 55); and
- active employees not yet fully eligible.

Costs would be fully accrued by the date the employee is fully eligible to receive benefits under the terms of the company-sponsored plan (the "full eligibility date").

Observation: *In the FASB's view, the full eligibility date concept is appropriate since further service need not be performed for the employee to receive full benefits. Typically, full eligibility is attained when an employee reaches a specific age and completes a specified period of service with the company (for example, 55 years of age and 10 years of service).*

Definition of the Obligation

In defining the obligation for postretirement benefits, the FASB has maintained certain concepts similar to pension accounting but has introduced new and modified terms designed specifically for postretirement benefits.

Accumulated postretirement benefit obligation (APBO). For retirees and their dependents and active employees fully eligible to receive benefits, the actuarial present value of benefits expected to be paid after retirement would be included in the APBO, along with a proportionate amount, based on employee service up to the measurement date, for active employees not yet fully eligible for postretirement benefits. The APBO is disclosed in the financial statements.

Expected postretirement benefit obligation (EPBO). The EPBO is the actuarial present value as of the measurement date of all benefits expected to be paid after retirement to employees and their dependents. It includes the APBO plus the actuarial present value of expected future service costs of active employees that have not yet reached the full eligibility date. The EPBO is not recorded or disclosed in the financial statements.

Observation: The only difference between the APBO and EPBO is the actuarial present value of expected future service costs of active employees not yet fully eligible for benefits.

Definition of Plan Assets

Consistent with pension accounting, plan assets would need to be segregated from the general assets of the company, restricted as to use (usually in a trust) and maintained exclusively for benefits payable or expected to be paid under the plan in order to reduce an employer's benefit obligation. (See chapter 11 for information relating to funding retiree health plans.)

Measurement

A single measurement approach would be required. Obligations would be accrued based on the following:

Attribution method. A benefit/years-of-service approach (generally referred to as the projected unit credit actuarial cost method) has been proposed to spread costs over accounting periods.

Observation: Because the Board found no compelling reason to switch from the approach used in pension accounting, it rejected the use of other actuarial approaches, including those under which costs are spread as a percentage of pay.

Attribution period. Costs generally would be spread ratably from date-of-hire (or credited service date if the plan grants credit only from a later date) to the full eligibility date, unless the plan's benefit formula specifies the benefits earned for full specific periods of service.

Observation: The FASB believes that if the terms of the plan specify a benefit formula, it would be consistent with pension accounting to follow that formula. However, the Board is aware that few retiree health plans today have such a benefit formula. Therefore, if no formula is specified, an approach consistent with pension accounting is stipulated. It is the FASB's objective that costs be spread over the period that the benefit is earned. This approach would record, in the Board's view, the proper balance sheet liability by the full eligibility date. After much deliberation, the Board rejected the concept of spreading costs over the entire service period (i.e., date-of-hire to the expected date of retirement), believing that the balance sheet liability would be understated at the full eligibility date because an employee could elect to retire with full benefits beginning with the full eligibility date. Moreover, the Board believes that costs should be recognized as benefits are "earned" and that no incremental benefits are "earned" for service beyond the full eligibility date.

Assumptions

Obligations would be measured using an explicit approach to assumptions that reflects the employer's best estimate of the plan's expected future experience with respect to each assumption, taking into account only current active and retired plan participants. Expected changes in the law and anticipated cost containment efforts or other plan amendments would not be anticipated in measuring the obligation or expense but would be accounted for as an actuarial gain or loss, or as a plan amendment, respectively, when they occur. Additional information on assumptions is provided in chapter 5.

The health care cost trend. The health care cost trend is defined as the estimate of the projected change in health care costs. The assumption as to the health care cost trend would be applied to current average per capita costs for retirees and would consider estimates of health care inflation, changes in health care utilization or delivery patterns, technological advances, and changes in the health status of plan participants. In selecting the health care cost trend rate, the ED recognizes that it may be appropriate to use different rates for different services (e.g., hospital care or dental services). The ED also recognizes that health care costs may not increase at a uniform rate over time.

Discount rate. The discount rate assumption would be based on the rates at which the benefits could be "effectively" settled. Employers could look to rates of return on high-quality, fixed-income investments currently available and expected to be available during the period the benefits are expected to be paid.

Other assumptions. Similar to pension accounting, assumptions concerning employee turnover, retirement age, mortality, and dependency status would be used to estimate the amount and timing of future retiree benefit payments.

Liability Recognition

A method of liability recognition is needed under any type of accrual accounting. Under the ED, annual expense would be computed first; the accrued liability reported in the balance sheet would then reflect the difference between the cumulative accrued expense and the actual amounts paid (or funded).

Minimum liability. Starting with fiscal years beginning after December 15, 1996 (for calendar year companies, the first quarter of 1997), the FASB proposes that companies record, as a minimum, a liability for postretirement benefits equal to the present value of the obligation expected to be paid to retirees and actives fully eligible, net of the fair value of plan assets, if any. If the accrued liability described above is less than this "minimum liability," an additional liability equal to the difference between the two would be recorded, offset by an intangible asset to the extent there are unrecognized prior service costs (including any unamortized transition obligation). Any additional amount would be charged to stockholder's equity (on a net of tax basis). Companies would determine annually any increase or decrease in the additional liability and intangible asset.

Observation: The annual increases or decreases under the minimum liability provisions would not affect a company's income statement.

Transition to Accrual Accounting

The obligation at the date the statement is adopted (the "transition obligation or asset") would be based on the APBO at that date, less any plan assets or accrued liabilities (assets) on the company's balance sheet.

Recognition. The ED proposes a single method for transition. The transition obligation would not be immediately recorded in the balance sheet or on the income statement, but it would be disclosed in the notes to the financial statements.

Observation: The Board considered immediate recognition of the postretirement benefit obligation but supported a prospective approach for practical reasons.

Amortization. The transition obligation would be amortized to expense over future years on a straight-line basis over the average remaining years of service (through expected date of retirement) of active employees expected to receive a benefit. However, under the ED, a company could elect to use 15 years if the computed period of amortization is less than 15 years. The FASB also proposes a requirement whereby additional amortization of the transition obligation would be recorded if the computed amortization on a cumulative basis is less than the amount that would have been recognized on a pay-as-you-go basis. This requirement is referred to as the "pay-as-you-go constraint."

Under the ED, the pay-as-you-go constraint would be operative in the following situations:

- Cumulative benefit payments subsequent to the transition date to fully eligible plan participants (retirees and actives) at the transition date exceed the sum of (1) the cumulative amortization of the entire transition obligation and (2) the cumulative interest on the unpaid transition obligation.

- Cumulative benefit payments subsequent to the transition date to all plan participants exceed the cumulative accrued postretirement benefit cost recognized subsequent to the transition date (including amounts required to be recognized pursuant to the preceding subparagraph).

An additional amount of the unamortized transition obligation would be recognized equal to the excess cumulative benefit payments in one or both of the above situations. For purposes of these tests, cumulative benefit payments would be reduced by any plan assets or any recognized accrued postretirement benefit obligation at the transition date.

Plan Amendments and Plan Initiation

Positive plan amendments (amendments that increase retiree health benefits) and plan initiation would generally be considered retroactive under the ED and would immediately increase the APBO. The increase in the APBO relating to retirees and actives would be amortized to expense over the remaining service period (to the full eligibility date) of active employees not yet fully eligible but expected to receive a benefit.

A reduction in the obligation due to a negative plan amendment (a plan amendment that reduces the retiree health benefit) would first be used to reduce any existing unrecognized prior service cost. Any remaining unamortized transition obligation would then be reduced. Any excess would be amortized over the remaining service period (to the full eligibility date) of active employees not yet fully eligible but expected to receive a benefit.

Components of Expense

The ED would require that an employer's postretirement benefit expense include a number of components. The ED refers to postretirement benefit cost rather than expense, because a portion of the cost in a period may be capitalized along with other costs as part of an asset such as inventory. However, consistent with common usage, "expense" is used for postretirement benefit cost in this book.

Service cost. The service cost component would be the increase in the APBO attributable to employee service for the period calculated using the beginning-of-the-year discount rate and the required attribution method.

Interest cost. The increase in the APBO attributable to the passage of time would be reflected in the interest cost component. It would be calculated by applying the beginning-of-the-year discount rate to the beginning-of-the-year APBO, adjusted for benefit payments to be made during the period.

Expected return on plan assets. For funded plans, the expected long-term earnings rate applied to the market-related value of the plan's assets, adjusted for contributions and benefit payments to be made during the period, would represent the expected return on plan assets (deducted from expense).

Prior service cost. This cost would be the amortization of retroactive benefits resulting from plan amendments and/or plan initiation that take place after the statement is adopted.

Gains and losses. This component would be the amortization of the unrecognized net gain or loss from previous periods. In general, gains and losses are changes in the APBO resulting from changes in assumptions or from experience different from that assumed. For funded plans, this component would also include the difference between the actual and expected return on plan assets. The ED would allow for prospective recognition of gains and losses. The minimum amount of amortization recognized in postretirement benefit expense for the period would be based on a "corridor approach" whereby a company could amortize only the portion of net accumulated gains and losses that exceeds 10 percent of the greater of the APBO or the market-related value of plan assets.

Companies would have the option of immediately recognizing gains and losses, provided that such a method is consistently applied. Gains not offsetting previously recognized losses would first be applied to reduce any unamortized transition obligation before being recognized in income.

Amortization of the transition obligation (or asset). As discussed previously, this component would represent the straight-line amortization of the transition obligation at the date the standard is adopted.

Using two hypothetical companies, figure 3.1 on page 29 illustrates the components of the APBO and the EPBO and figure 3.2 on page 30 compares the components of expense in the first year under accrual accounting to pay-as-you-go amounts. Actual measurement of an employer's obligation and expense will vary depending on a number of factors, including the terms of the plan, demographics, and assumptions. In the hypothetical examples, the company with a "mature" population has a few active employees per retiree, and the company with an immature population has relatively more active employees per retiree.

Accounting for Settlements

As in pension accounting, a settlement would be defined as a transaction that:

- is an irrevocable action;
- relieves the employer of primary responsibility for a postretirement benefit obligation; and
- eliminates significant risks related to the obligation and the assets used to effect the settlement.

When a settlement occurs, companies would immediately recognize deferred gains and losses, except that settlement gains would first be offset against the remaining unamortized transition obligation. There would otherwise be no acceleration of the unamortized transition obligation or of unrecognized prior service costs.

FIGURE 3.1   Illustration of Benefit Obligations

**Company A: Mature Population
(In Millions)**

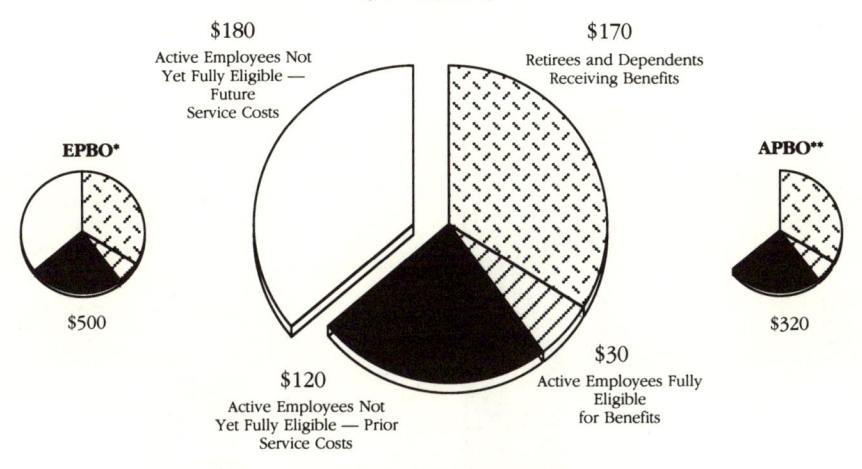

$180 Active Employees Not Yet Fully Eligible — Future Service Costs

$170 Retirees and Dependents Receiving Benefits

EPBO* $500

APBO** $320

$120 Active Employees Not Yet Fully Eligible — Prior Service Costs

$30 Active Employees Fully Eligible for Benefits

**Company B: Immature Population
(In Millions)**

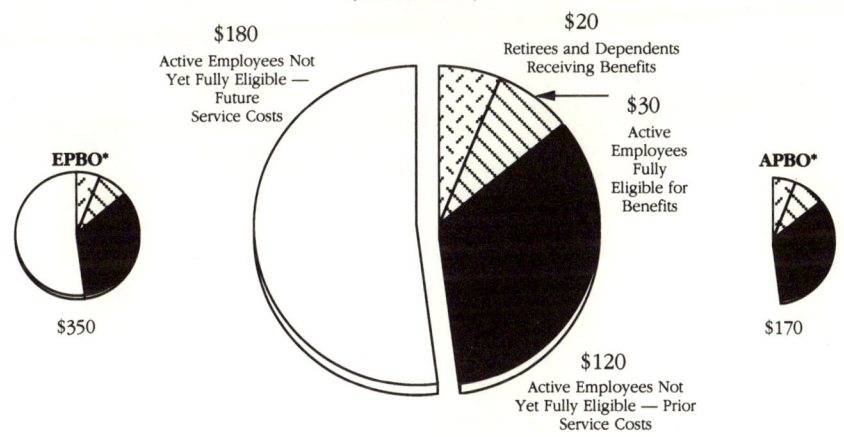

$180 Active Employees Not Yet Fully Eligible — Future Service Costs

$20 Retirees and Dependents Receiving Benefits

$30 Active Employees Fully Eligible for Benefits

EPBO* $350

APBO* $170

$120 Active Employees Not Yet Fully Eligible — Prior Service Costs

* Expected Postretirement Benefit Obligation
** Accumulated Postretirement Benefit Obligation

FIGURE 3.2 Components of Expense under Accrual Accounting Compared to Pay-As-You-Go — Year of Adoption

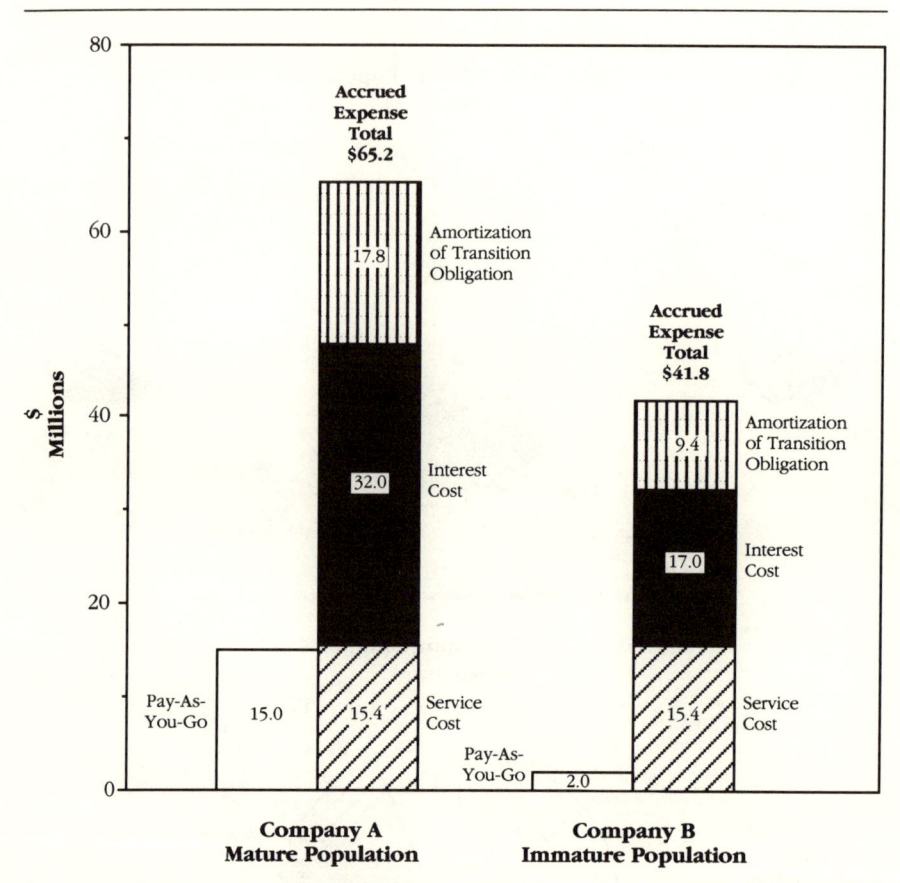

[Bar chart showing $ Millions on y-axis from 0 to 80.

Company A — Mature Population:
- Pay-As-You-Go: 15.0
- Accrued Expense Total $65.2:
  - Service Cost: 15.4
  - Interest Cost: 32.0
  - Amortization of Transition Obligation: 17.8

Company B — Immature Population:
- Pay-As-You-Go: 2.0
- Accrued Expense Total $41.8:
  - Service Cost: 15.4
  - Interest Cost: 17.0
  - Amortization of Transition Obligation: 9.4]

Accounting for Curtailments

A curtailment is defined as an event that significantly reduces the expected years of future service of current employees or eliminates the accrual of benefits for some or all of the future service of a significant number of active plan participants. Typical situations include reductions in work force or plan suspensions or terminations that result in elimination of future benefit accruals for some or all employees.

When the occurrence of a curtailment is probable and the dollar effect can be reasonably estimated, a company would be required to compute a net gain or loss. Net losses would be recognized in earnings when the occurrence of a curtailment is probable and the net effect is estimable; net gains would be recognized when the related employees terminate or when the plan amendment or suspension is adopted. The ED provides the computational requirements for determining the net gain or loss in a curtailment; basically, the net gain or loss is the sum of the following two items:

- a gain or loss computed as the portion of unrecognized prior service costs (arising from any remaining unamortized transition obligation or the cost of retroactive plan amendments) that relate to years of service no longer expected to be rendered; and
- a gain or loss computed as the net change in the APBO resulting from the event; however, this net change must first be offset against any existing unrecognized net gain or loss.

Other Accounting Issues

The ED proposes guidance in the accounting for other aspects of postretirement benefits. Generally, the accounting rules proposed are similar to those in pension accounting.

Business combinations. In amending APB Opinion No. 16, the ED would provide guidance concerning the treatment of postretirement benefits in a business combination accounted for under the purchase method. The assignment of the purchase price to individual assets acquired and liabilities assumed would include a liability for the APBO in excess of the fair value of the plan assets at the date of purchase. The measurement of the APBO at the date of purchase would reflect the purchaser's assumptions and the elimination of any previously existing unrecognized net gain or loss, unrecognized prior service cost, and unamortized transition obligation for the acquired employer's plan.

Non-U.S. postretirement plans. The only special consideration with regard to non-U.S. plans is that the effective date with regard to these plans would be delayed two years to 1994.

Employers with two or more plans. Unfunded plans may be aggregated for measurement purposes if the plans provide different benefits to the same group of employees or if the plans provide the same benefits to different groups of employees. Funded plans would not be aggregated with unfunded plans for measurement purposes. In terms of disclosure, overfunded plans would not be aggregated with underfunded plans and retiree health plans would be shown separately from other retiree welfare plans.

Multiemployer plans. A multiemployer plan is defined as a plan to which two or more unrelated employers contribute, usually pursuant to collective bargaining agreements. The expense recognized would be the required contribution to the plan for the period.

Measurement date. A company would be permitted to select any date up to three months prior to its balance sheet date to perform measurements of its obligation (and related plan assets) for postretirement benefits.

Special termination benefits. Employers would recognize an expense when employees accept the offer of special termination and the amount can be reasonably estimated.

Amendment to APB Opinion No. 12. Under APB Opinion No. 12, individual deferred compensation contracts that are not equivalent to pension plans (and therefore not covered by SFAS No. 87) are generally accrued for over the period of active employment from the date the contract is executed to the expected retirement date. The ED would amend this provision of APB Opinion No. 12 by requiring that deferred compensation contracts be accrued in accordance with the terms of the individual contracts. If terms are not specified, the contracts would be accrued for from the date the contract is executed to the date the employee attains full eligibility for the contractual benefits.

Disclosure

The Board proposes the following disclosures for defined postretirement benefit plans:

- a description of the plan or plans, including the employee groups covered, types of benefits provided, funding policy, and types of assets held;
- the components of expense;
- the funded status reconciliation;
- the assumed discount rate;
- the weighted-average assumed health care cost trend rate;

- the effect on the APBO and net periodic postretirement benefit cost of either a one percentage point increase or decrease in the health care cost trend rate; and
- the "vested" postretirement benefit obligation, defined as a measure of the employer's obligation assuming all active employees eligible to receive any benefits terminated immediately.

Effective Date and Public Comments

Recognizing the need for a long period in which companies can develop the data and systems needed to measure their benefit obligation and expense under accrual accounting, the FASB proposes delayed effective dates. The proposed statement would be effective for fiscal years beginning after December 15, 1991 (i.e., accrual accounting would begin no later than the first quarter of fiscal 1992). Small nonpublic employers (under 100 participants) and foreign plans would have until the first quarter of fiscal 1994 to adopt the statement. Application of the "minimum liability" requirement would be delayed until 1997. Earlier adoption would be encouraged.

The FASB has designated a six-month period, ending August 14, 1989, during which individuals and organizations may submit written comments on this project to the FASB Director of Research and Technical Activities. Additionally, the FASB will conduct public hearings to obtain information from and views of interested parties about the standards proposed in the ED. The hearings are scheduled for October 10-12, 1989 at the Grand Hyatt Hotel in New York and November 2-3, 1989 at the J.W. Marriott in Washington, D.C.

Adopting Accrual Accounting Now

After analyzing the specific impact that accrual accounting may have on its financial position, some companies may consider adopting accrual accounting before the proposed requirements are issued in a final statement. Current accounting as described in FASB TB 87-1 allows companies to begin to accrue prospectively or to recognize their full postretirement benefit obligation immediately if they elect to switch to accrual accounting. Under the ED, the TB would be rescinded effective with the issuance of the final standard. Consequently, companies selecting the immediate recognition option would need to change their accounting policy before the final statement is issued.

Observation: Companies considering immediate recognition — perhaps those that would be reversing significant deferred tax credits into income when adopting SFAS No. 96 — would generally have higher expense under accrual accounting than under pay-as-you-go.

Employers electing to recognize the current unrecognized accumulated obligation by recording a cumulative catch-up adjustment in the income statement in the period of change face an issue unresolved at the time of this writing. To record the unrecognized obligation currently under the TB entails adoption of a policy of recognizing gains and losses as well as prior service costs immediately in the period incurred. One of the more significant unresolved issues centers on whether an employer who adopts accrual accounting early using an immediate recognition approach will have latitude to elect delayed recognition of gains and losses when the FASB issues its final statement. The FASB may specifically address this issue in the final statement.

TABLE 3.1 Comparison Between FASB Exposure Draft on Postretirement Benefits and SFAS Nos. 87 and 88

Issue	FASB Exposure Draft	Statement 87/88 Approach
Accrual accounting	Costs would be accrued during an employee's working career. Cash basis (pay-as-you-go) and terminal accrual (accrue at retirement) methods would be prohibited.	Same.
Flexibility	Companies would follow a single measurement approach.	Same.
Attribution (actuarial cost) approach	A benefit/years-of-service approach would be required (projected unit credit actuarial cost method).	Same.
Attribution period	If the plan contains a formula that defines (or bases) benefits on specific years of service, companies would be required to follow that formula. If there is no formula, benefits would be spread ratably from the date of hire to the *full eligibility date*. Attribution period would begin at the date of hire unless the plan's benefit formula defines a later date as the beginning of the credited service period.	Attribution period is based on the formula inherent in the plan contract which, for most pension plans, is virtually the entire service period.
Discounting	The obligation would be discounted to a present value.	Same.
Assumptions	An *explicit approach* would be required.	Same.

NOTE: The *italicized* terms are defined in the glossary of terms, box 3.1.

TABLE 3.1 Comparison Between FASB Exposure Draft on Postretirement Benefits and SFAS Nos. 87 and 88 (continued)

Issue	FASB Exposure Draft	Statement 87/88 Approach
Projection of benefits	For retiree health benefits, costs would be projected based on current per capita retiree claims costs (gross claims) with recognition of Medicare reimbursement rate based on current law. Other benefits would be projected based on plan formula.	Benefits are projected based on the formula inherent in the plan, using a salary progression (future salary increases) assumption.
Heath care inflation assumption	A *health care cost trend rate* would be applied to gross claims to project future health care costs. Future changes in the law (e.g. Medicare) and in the plan would not be anticipated in setting the cost trend rate.	This issue is not applicable to pension plans.
Discount rate assumption	A settlement rate assumption would be required. However, because it is generally not possible to currently settle the health care obligation, employers could look to rates on high-quality, fixed-income investments.	A settlement rate is required (i.e., current rate at which the obligation could be effectively settled). Employers could look to annuity rates, Pension Benefit Guaranty Corporation rates, or rates on high-quality, fixed-income investments.
Other assumptions	Other assumptions would include turnover, retirement age, mortality, and dependent status.	Other assumptions include turnover, retirement age and mortality.

TABLE 3.1 Comparison Between FASB Exposure Draft on Postretirement Benefits and SFAS Nos. 87 and 88 (continued)

Issue	FASB Exposure Draft	Statement 87/88 Approach
Actuarial gains and losses	Immediate or delayed recognition would be allowed but must be consistently applied. If immediate recognition is chosen, gains (losses) would be first offset against any unamortized transition obligation (asset). If delayed recognition is selected, a corridor approach would be required as a minimum. Under this approach, the minimum amortization would be the unrecognized net gain or loss in excess of 10% of the greater of the *accumulated postretirement benefit obligation (APBO)* or the market-related value of plan assets amortized over the average remaining service period to expected retirement of employees expected to receive benefits.	Same, except under option of immediate recognition gains and losses are not offset against any unamortized transition obligation or asset.
Plan assets	Plan assets would be segregated and restricted solely to pay the benefits provided under the plan.	Same.

TABLE 3.1 Comparison Between FASB Exposure Draft on Postretirement Benefits and SFAS Nos. 87 and 88 (continued)

Issue	FASB Exposure Draft	Statement 87/88 Approach
Market-related value of assets	Expense is measured either by the market-related value (smoothed value of plan assets over period not to exceed five years) or fair value; fair value is required for balance sheet and financial statement disclosure.	Same.
Plan initiation and amendments—measuring the obligation	Initiations or amendments would be considered to be retroactive (generally a prior service obligation would be created or eliminated) unless new/amended benefits are earned only for future service.	Defined by plan.
Plan initiation and amendments—measuring expense	Unless the plan participants are all or almost all retirees, prior service cost relating to both retirees and active employees would be deferred and amortized over remaining service to full eligibility date of active employees expected to receive benefits. Negative amendments would be first offset against unrecognized prior service cost or unamortized *transition obligation,* with remainder (if any) amortized in same fashion as positive amendments.	Unless the plan participants are all or almost all retirees, prior service cost relating to both retirees and active employees is deferred and amortized over remaining service of active employees expected to receive benefits. Negative amendments first offset against unrecognized prior service cost with remainder (if any) recognized in same fashion as positive amendments.

TABLE 3.1 Comparison Between FASB Exposure Draft on Postretirement Benefits and SFAS Nos. 87 and 88 (continued)

Issue	FASB Exposure Draft	Statement 87/88 Approach
Transition—measurement	The transition obligation (asset) would be measured as the APBO at the date the statement is adopted less the fair value of plan assets and any accrued liabilities (assets) on the company's balance sheet.	The transition obligation (asset) is measured as the projected benefit obligation at the date statement is adopted less the fair value of plan assets and any accrued liabilities (assets) on a company's balance sheet.
Transition—recognizing expense	A prospective approach would be required—the transition obligation would not be recorded on the balance sheet; it would be amortized to expense using the straight-line method over the average remaining service period to the date of expected retirement of active employees expected to receive benefits under the plan. If the average remaining service period is less than 15 years, 15 years may be used at the company's option.	Same.
Pay-as-you-go constraint	In addition to the required amortization, the amortization of the transition obligation must be no less rapid than under pay-as-you-go. Under this constraint, additional amortization would be recorded to the extent that ☐ cumulative benefit payments to all plan participants exceed the cumulative	No similar requirement under SFAS No. 87.

TABLE 3.1 Comparison Between FASB Exposure Draft on Postretirement Benefits and SFAS Nos. 87 and 88 (continued)

Issue	FASB Exposure Draft	Statement 87/88 Approach
	expense (subsequent to adoption); and	
	☐ cumulative benefit payments to employees who were retired or fully eligible for benefits at the transition date exceed the sum of cumulative amortization of the entire transition obligation plus the cumulative interest on the unpaid transition obligation (both from date of adoption).	
	Cumulative benefit payments would be reduced by any plan assets or accrued liabilities at the transition date.	
Balance sheet recognition	An *accrued liability* would be recognized equal to cumulative expense less benefits paid (or funded). Under a *minimum liability* provision, a liability equal to the actuarial present value of the obligation expected to be paid to retirees and fully eligible active employees would need to be reflected. If this minimum liability is greater than the accrued liability, an additional liability would be recorded, generally offset by an intangible asset.	Similar except minimum liability is based on accumulated benefit obligation (with no salary progression).

TABLE 3.1 Comparison Between FASB Exposure Draft on Postretirement Benefits and SFAS Nos. 87 and 88 (continued)

Issue	FASB Exposure Draft	Statement 87/88 Approach
Effective date of new standard	☐ Accrual accounting provisions would be effective for fiscal years beginning after 12/15/91 (first quarter of fiscal 1992). ☐ Requirements relating to foreign plans and small employers would be effective for fiscal years beginning after 12/15/93 (first quarter of fiscal 1994). ☐ Minimum liability requirements would be effective for fiscal years beginning after 12/15/96 (first quarter of fiscal 1997).	The new standard was generally effective two years after issuance. Requirements relating to minimum liability, small employers, and foreign plans were effective two years later.
Purchase business combination	Acquiring company would be required to establish a liability or asset in the purchase price allocation, based on the difference between APBO and fair value of plan assets at date of purchase, but the measurement would be based on the acquiring company's assumptions.	Acquiring company is required to establish a liability or asset in the purchase price allocation, based on the difference between projected benefit obligation and fair value of plan assets at date of purchase.
Disclosures	☐ Similar to disclosures called for in SFAS No. 87. ☐ Weight-average health care cost trend assumption. ☐ Sensitivity analysis (1 percentage point	☐ Description of plan including funding policy, employee groups covered, benefits provided, benefit formula and types of assets held. ☐ *Components of expense.*

TABLE 3.1 Comparison Between FASB Exposure Draft on Postretirement Benefits and SFAS Nos. 87 and 88 (continued)

Issue	FASB Exposure Draft	Statement 87/88 Approach
	change in health care cost trend rate). ☐ Component of expense relating to amortization of transition amount. ☐ *Vested postretirement benefit obligation* (actuarial present value of obligation for retirees and active employees assuming they retired or terminated immediately).	☐ Funded status (plan obligations less the fair value of plan assets) reconciled to amounts reported in balance sheet. ☐ Key assumptions. ☐ Vested benefit obligation (actuarial present value of legally vested benefits).
More than one plan	Company can elect to account for related groups of plans unless a plan is funded. Health plan measurement and disclosures would be separate from those for other plans.	Each plan must be accounted for separately – (e.g., qualified funded pension plan accounted for separately from unqualified unfunded supplementary pension benefit plans). Disclosure for overfunded plans separate from underfunded plans.
Multiemployer plans	Expense as payments are due.	Same.
Defined contribution plans	Expense as contributions are due. Accrue during working career if contributions are required after the retirement date.	Same.
Measurement date	Any date within three months of company's year end.	Same.

TABLE 3.1 Comparison Between FASB Exposure Draft on Postretirement Benefits and SFAS Nos. 87 and 88 (continued)

Issue	FASB Exposure Draft	Statement 87/88 Approach
Settlements of the obligation (i.e., complete transfer of risk outside the company)	Same as SFAS No. 88, except settlement gain would be first offset against unamortized transition obligation.	Immediately recognize deferred gains and losses and transition assets; no acceleration of deferred prior service costs or transition obligation.
Curtailments (i.e., reduction in workforce or complete elimination of future benefit accruals for some or all employees)	Immediately recognize deferred prior service cost or transition obligation; no acceleration of deferred gains and losses or transition asset.	Same.
Special termination benefits	Similar to SFAS No. 88 except that incremental cost of termination would be immediately expensed; effect of change in expected retirement date would be deferred as an actuarial loss.	Expense when employees accept the offer and the amount can be reasonably estimated.

BOX 3.1 Glossary of Terms

Accrued liability. Liability representing the difference between the cumulative expense and amounts funded or paid by the employer.

Accumulated postretirement benefit obligation (APBO). The actuarial present value of benefits expected to be paid after retirement that can be attributed to employee service up to the measurement date. The calculation of the APBO includes benefits expected to be paid to retirees, active employees fully eligible, and a proportionate amount for active employees not yet fully eligible for benefits.

Attribution period. The period over which costs would be accrued for active employees not yet fully eligible.

Components of expense. The components of net periodic postretirement benefit cost would include

- service cost—the increase in APBO for current service;
- interest cost—the increase in APBO attributable to the accrual of interest on the obligation;
- expected return on plan assets (funded plans);
- amortization of transition obligation or asset; and
- amortization of gains and losses and prior service costs.

Discount rate. The rate at which the obligation would be effectively settled. Employers could select a rate reflecting the pretax rates of return available at each measurement date for high-quality, fixed-income investments that will mature over approximately the same periods as expected benefit payments.

Explicit approach to assumptions. An approach under which each significant assumption used reflects the best estimate of the plan's future experience solely with respect to that assumption.

Full eligibility date. The date that employees have met age and/or service requirements to qualify for all of the benefits they are expected to receive under the plan.

Health care cost trend rate. An assumption about future changes in the cost of the health care benefits currently provided by the plan due to factors other than demographics of the plan participants (e.g., health care inflation, changes in health care utilization or delivery patterns, technological advances, and changes in the health status of plan participants).

Minimum liability. The unfunded APBO only for retirees and actives fully eligible.

Transition obligation (asset). The APBO, net of any plan assets and balance sheet accruals, at the date the standard is adopted.

Vested postretirement benefit obligation. The actuarial present value at the measurement date of the benefits expected to be paid to retirees, former employees, and active employees assuming they retired or terminated immediately. This term has sometimes been referred to as the "walk-away benefit obligation."

4

The Field Test: The Companies, Their Plans, the Measurement Process, and Implementation Problems

The FERF, in recognition of the evolving nature of accounting for retiree health benefits, sponsored this Field Test. The purpose of the Field Test is to assist the FASB and other interested parties in assessing the potential impact of the proposed accounting standard as it relates to retiree health benefits and to identify measurement and implementation issues that may affect compliance with a new standard. The FERF and Coopers & Lybrand agreed that the study would be limited to retiree health benefits because the measurement of these benefits is generally more complex and raises many more data and implementation problems than other postretirement benefits, such as life insurance.

This chapter provides comparative information regarding the Field Test companies and their plans and discusses the methodology used to estimate the obligation and expense for each company. In addition, it summarizes implementation and data problems encountered during the Field Test.

Because of the importance of maintaining the anonymity of the Field Test companies, certain information that could lead to identification of any particular company has been omitted. For example, any plan provisions that may be particularly unusual, or company information that could lead to identification is not included in the Field Test.

The Field Test Companies

Twenty-five major U.S. companies participated in the Field Test. However, in certain cases, divisions or subsidiaries of a company were considered as a separate company for purposes of reporting certain Field Test results. In addition, for a number of companies only selected divisions or subsidiaries participated. The companies are located in all parts of the United States and a number of them had foreign plans which were not considered in the Field Test. Manufacturing, banking, oil, and a number of other industries are represented. Each of the Field Test companies had total revenue in 1988 in excess of $250 million, with most over $1 billion.

In addition, the companies vary greatly in demographic composition. Table 4.1 shows the active to retiree ratio of the participating companies. Dependents were not included in calculating this ratio.

TABLE 4.1 Active to Retiree Ratio of Participating Companies

Definition	Ratio of Active Employees to Retirees	Number of Companies
Highly mature	Less than two actives per retiree	9
Mature	Two to six actives per retiree	13
Immature	More than six actives per retiree	4
		26

Observation: *Since only a few participating companies are immature, results shown in chapter 6 relating to the immature group may not be representative of a wider sample of immature companies.*

While the majority of the companies were large with a significant number of retirees, a few companies with a smaller number of retirees (with less than 2,000 retirees and dependents) participated. Approximately 1,000,000 retirees and dependents of retirees are currently participants in the Field Test companies' plans.

The Plans

Generally, under the ED separate plans would be measured separately. However, an employer may aggregate data from unfunded plans for measurement purposes if: (a) those plans provide different benefits to the same group of employees, or (b) those plans provide the same benefits to different groups of employees. However, this definition raises a number of questions. For example, should an HMO be combined with an indemnity arrangement if offered to some retirees? If a company has numerous employee groups, each offered a slightly different retiree health benefit, should these plans be combined or measured separately? Generally, for retiree health benefits, the term "plan" is not as clearly defined as for pensions. Companies often use the term plan to differentiate between types of health benefits offered, the period such benefits are payable, the level of retiree contributions, the year of retirement, as well as other factors. For purposes of the Field Test, the definition of what constituted a plan was generally left to the companies and what they perceived to be separate plans. For example, a number of companies wanted obligation and expense measured separately for different groups of employees (e.g., hourly and salaried), even if the benefits offered differed slightly or not at all. Of course, where plan provisions significantly affected cost (e.g., deductible amounts or out-of-pocket maximums), those provisions were taken into account.[1]

Eligibility

Almost all of the participating companies provided coverage for the life of the retiree.

Spousal coverage was typically continued for life unless the retiree died. In this event, many of the companies terminated the surviving spouse's coverage if he or she remarried, or after a certain period of time such as six months to a year. In a number of instances, coverage was continued on a fully contributory basis.

The majority of the Field Test plans provided dependent coverage for children; typically until age 18 or 19 unless the dependent child was a full-time student. Then coverage would typically be continued until age 23 or 25.

All of the companies have early retirement provisions whereby employees retiring from the company prior to age 65 would be eligible for health benefits. Coverage for these early retirees and their dependents almost always is a continuation of their benefit coverage as active employees.

Most early retirement provisions allowed employees to retire at age 55, with 10 or 15 years of service. A number of the companies' plans provided for early retirement once an employee reached a combination of age and service that equaled a certain number; for example, age plus years of service would be equal to 75 or 80.

HMOs

A number of the Field Test companies do not offer HMOs to their retirees. Those that do generally have a very low retiree HMO participation rate.

Deductibles, Maximums, and Coinsurance

The Field Test plans varied in annual deductible amounts, annual employee out-of-pocket and lifetime maximums, as well as required retiree contributions. Annual deductibles for the medical plans ranged from approximately $50 to $300 for single and $100 to $600 for family coverage. Moreover, dental and prescription drug plans typically required that separate deductibles or copayments be satisfied.

Most of the plans did not have annual plan maximums, but limited annual retiree out-of-pocket costs. Annual out-of-pocket maximums ranged from less than $500 to $4,000. Most of the plans had annual individual out-of-pocket maximums in the $1,000 to $2,000 range. Lifetime maximums ranged from less than $100,000 to more than $1,000,000 with a number of plans providing unlimited coverage for life. A number of companies had different lifetime maximums apply before and after age 65.

Observation: The ED would require that the current lifetime maximum described in a plan be assumed to remain constant (i.e., the maximum would not be raised by the anticipated increases in future cost) unless the plan specifically included increases. As costs are inflated or trended forward and lifetime maximums remain at current levels, an effective cap would be placed on a company's obligation and expense. However, a number of the Field Test companies have annual reinstatement of maximums or some other reinstatement (such as full lifetime maximum with evidence of insurability). This kind of provision in a plan may effectively make the lifetime maximums inoperative and it may be appropriate to ignore them in measuring obligation and expense.

Approximately 60 percent of the companies required a monthly retiree contribution toward the cost of health coverage. Retiree contributions were generally much lower for the over 65 retiree group. A number of the companies based the required contribution on a constant percentage of costs, while others required a fixed-dollar contribution.

Nearly all of the plans required retiree coinsurance on some or all services. Coinsurance generally ranged from 0 percent to 20 percent, with some plans requiring 50 percent coinsurance for certain coverage such as psychiatric care.

Medicare

One of the key factors in determining a company's costs for its retiree health plans is the manner in which it integrates payments with Medicare. Once a retired individual reaches age 65, Medicare generally becomes the primary payer. There are basically three methods by which companies can integrate their payments for retiree health benefits with Medicare: carve-out, coordination of benefits (COB), and exclusion. Carve-out is the integration method that is the least costly for the employer and coordination is the most costly. (See chapter 10 for a more complete description of the three methods.) Table 4.2 shows the percentage of plans utilizing each method. The numbers shown are not inclusive of all Field Test Company plans, as a number of plans are offered only to retirees under age 65. Also, the integration methods did not apply to certain other plans.

TABLE 4.2

Medicare Integration Method	Percentage
Carve-out	59%
Exclusion	24
Coordination	17

Approximately 25 percent of the companies pay the Medicare Part B premium ($24.80 in 1988 and $27.90 in 1989). A number of those that do pay the premium capped the amount at something less than the full premium. Many of the companies that paid the Part B premium for retirees also paid the Part B premium for eligible spouses.

Other Coverage

Approximately one-third of the Field Test companies provide dental coverage, and only a few provide vision coverage. Nearly all of the participating companies provide a prescription drug benefit as part of their indemnity arrangements. In addition, a number provided a stand-alone prescription drug benefit, usually utilizing a mail order prescription drug company.

The Measurement Process

An actuarial valuation is designed to make the best estimate of future benefit payments and their present value based on actuarial assumptions concerning future events. In estimating future benefits, it is first necessary to estimate who will be eligible to receive benefits each year—the covered retiree group—and the average per capita cost of each future year's health care benefits.

The valuation of retiree health benefits is a more complex process than a typical pension actuarial valuation, mainly because:

- The utilization of health care varies greatly by individual, and patterns of usage may change over time, making it difficult to estimate average per capita costs by age. Moreover, this is complicated by such factors as lifetime maximums and average per capita deductible amounts.

- Benefit payments will be influenced by a number of factors that are difficult to predict such as the level of health care costs at the time services are delivered in the future, dependents who will be covered under the plan, and the availability of primary coverage from alternative sources. In particular, it is difficult to predict the effect of non-price factors on health care costs such as intensity and technology.

- The measurement of retiree health benefits is a developing practice. There is little consensus on how to measure these obligations and how to select actuarial assumptions necessary to calculate these obligations. As a result, cost estimates can vary depending on the methodology and actuarial assumptions used.

Numerous problems were encountered in developing a methodology for the Field Test and then implementing that methodology for 25 companies that had very different plans, demographics, and medical claims data. The most significant implementation issues are addressed in this report—many others are not, due to space considerations. The detailed methodology developed for the Field Test was designed to identify data and implementation problems and to provide the companies with underlying information related to their costs. Of course, the measurement of retiree health benefits is in an evolutionary stage and work will still need to be done to find practical solutions to some of these issues. In the future, additional methods and procedures will be developed and tested that may make the measurement process less difficult.

The Field Test Methodology—Overview

Detailed information from each of the participating companies regarding their plans, the demographic composition of their employee and retiree populations, and their medical claims experience was obtained from each company. To summarize, the following four steps were taken to provide each company with a retiree health valuation as of the assumed date of adoption of accrual accounting under the ED (January 1, 1988).

- Determine the retiree health benefit coverage—Current benefit plan materials that explain existing coverage were catalogued and reviewed with each company to understand what benefits are currently being offered.

☐ Analyze claims and demographic data—Information regarding current benefit recipients (i.e., retirees and dependents) and claims experience was examined using the company's internal records and those of its health insurers or plan administrators. From this information, average per capita costs for a one-year period were identified—the "baseline costs" generally broken down by age, sex, status (dependent/retiree), and health care service sectors for the indemnity plans. In addition, other breakdowns were provided where appropriate (e.g., by type of benefits and delivery systems such as HMOs and PPOs).

☐ Select actuarial assumptions—Economic research on trends in health care costs and the relation of health care to general inflation was performed to provide basic data to the Field Test companies on the selection of a range of health care cost trend assumptions. Each company then selected appropriate cost trend assumptions which, along with demographic assumptions as to anticipated employee turnover, mortality, early retirement, marital status, etc., form the basis for estimating future benefit payments. A discount rate assumption was also selected which was then applied to determine each company's obligation as of the date of adoption.

☐ Project obligations and expense—Using the methodology in the ED, obligations and expense were estimated for the year of adoption and future years based on the baseline costs and assumptions described above. In addition, alternative estimates of obligations and expense were projected to show the sensitivity to changes in the health care cost trend and discount rate assumptions and the impact of using alternative accounting approaches.

Each Field Test company was provided with a detailed actuarial report which served as the basis for this consolidated report.

The remainder of this chapter contains a more detailed discussion of the methodology used to develop baseline costs and to perform the actuarial valuations, and also discusses some of the data problems and measurement issues encountered.

Estimating Baseline Costs—The Use of Plan, Demographic, and Claims Information

For purposes of the Field Test, the estimation of each company's obligation for retiree health benefits generally began with the identification of average per capita costs for a one-year period. This starting point was called "baseline cost." Under the ED, estimated average per capita cost is treated as an assumption. For purposes of the Field Test, average per capita costs were estimated taking into account such items as the amount and probability of future claims.

Because of the nature of the Field Test, detailed information was requested from each participating company relating to medical claims, eligibility information, and plan design. Claims tapes were received, in most cases from the companies' insurance carriers, as well as eligibility tapes and plan information, such as Summary Plan Descriptions (SPDs) and relevant internal memos.

Eligible Charges vs. Incurred Claims

To understand the discussion of baseline cost presented in this chapter, it is important to differentiate between "eligible charges" and "incurred claims." Eligible charges generally represent the gross amount of the bills for services provided to retirees. Incurred claims are eligible charges less retiree copayments and deductibles, other insurance payments, and Medicare payments. In other words, incurred claims represent the net amount paid by the employer prior to recognition of retiree contributions, if any. Figure 4.1 illustrates this concept.

FIGURE 4.1 Eligible Charges to Incurred Claims

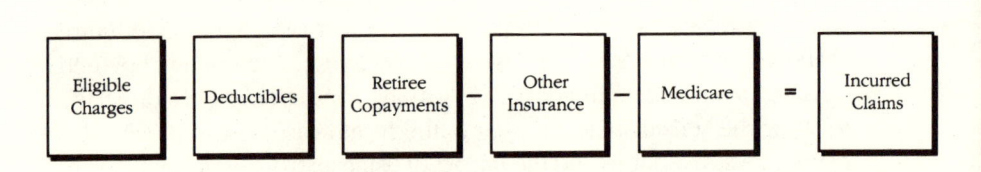

Eligible Charges − Deductibles − Retiree Copayments − Other Insurance − Medicare = Incurred Claims

In the past, actuarial valuations have generally been based on a projection of incurred claims cost. (The health care cost trend assumption was applied to the net cost.) To insure consistency of the Field Test approach with the guidance in the ED, however, the cost trend assumptions were applied to the gross eligible charges (by service sector) and copayments, other insurance and Medicare payments were projected separately. However, for many of the companies, Medicare payment information was not available. For these companies, eligible charges were considered to be net of Medicare payments.

Observation: *If the health care cost trend was applied to incurred claims, it would have implicitly assumed that the deductible and any plan maximum amounts would have risen proportionately, which would not satisfy the ED requirement that changes in plan terms cannot be anticipated before they actually are adopted.*

Since costs associated with different health care services may increase at different rates, eligible charges were grouped by type of service for use in developing future average per capita incurred claims costs. Based on a Health Care Financing Administration (HCFA) model used to project national health care expenditures, six categories of health service sectors were identified. The research and findings relating to the six service sectors and health care cost trends are further discussed in chapter 5.

Figures 4.2 and 4.3 illustrate how 1986 eligible charges were analyzed by service sector before and after Medicare payments had been taken into account. Information presented is based on combined data from a number of Field Test companies.

Observation: Analyzing claims based on health care service sector provided valuable information for many of the Field Test companies. As discussed in chapter 5, health care cost trends were selected by the companies for each health care service sector. In addition, companies considering certain cost management techniques would be able to analyze the effectiveness of certain options based on the most significant portion of their costs. For example, it is interesting to note that prescription drug costs were a substantial portion of eligible charges after Medicare was taken into account. However, the figures shown do not take into account the expanded drug coverage provided by the Medicare Catastrophic Coverage Act (see chapter 9 for additional information).

For the Field Test, the components of baseline cost were generally based on 1986 information. Total dollar amounts used to derive total 1986 incurred claim costs were broken down by eligible charges (by health care service sector), deductibles, copayments, and Medicare payments. These costs were then separately captured by age, sex, and status and expressed as average per capita amounts.

Observation: In estimating average per capita costs, it would have been preferable to analyze medical claims data for more than one year. Utilizing more extensive data may provide better estimates as data anomalies or experience trends may more easily be observed. However, as discussed later in this chapter, the claims data needed for valuing retiree health benefit programs has not traditionally been maintained by or for companies. For this reason, it was generally not feasible to utilize more than 12 to 18 months of claims experience for purposes of the Field Test.

54 *Retiree Health Benefits*

FIGURE 4.2 Eligible Charges by Service Sector—Pre-Medicare

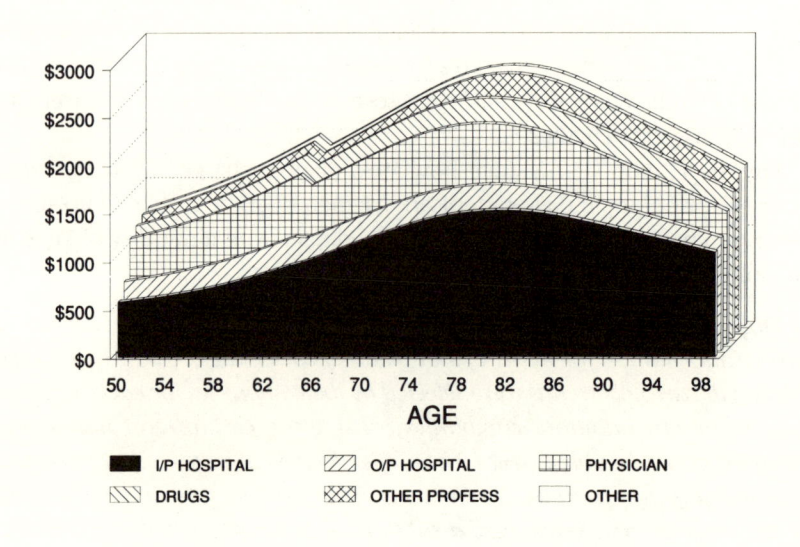

FIGURE 4.3 Eligible Charges by Service Sector—Post-Medicare

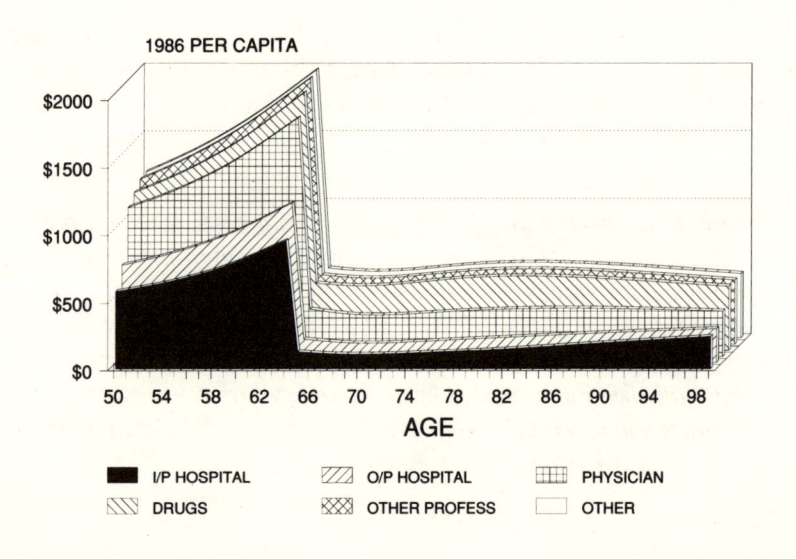

Adjusting for Fluctuations in Claims Cost

Per capita claims cost in certain age brackets may show "spikes" of high costs due to high claims for one or two individuals and a relatively small number of retirees in these age brackets. While it is expected that spikes may occur in future years as well, it may happen at different ages. Accordingly, using an actuarial technique called graduation, each component of average per capita incurred claims for 1986 was graduated or "smoothed" to get a realistic average cost at each age.

Figure 4.4 illustrates the effect of this graduation process on one company's inpatient hospital charges.

FIGURE 4.4 Inpatient Hospital—Raw Data vs. Graduated

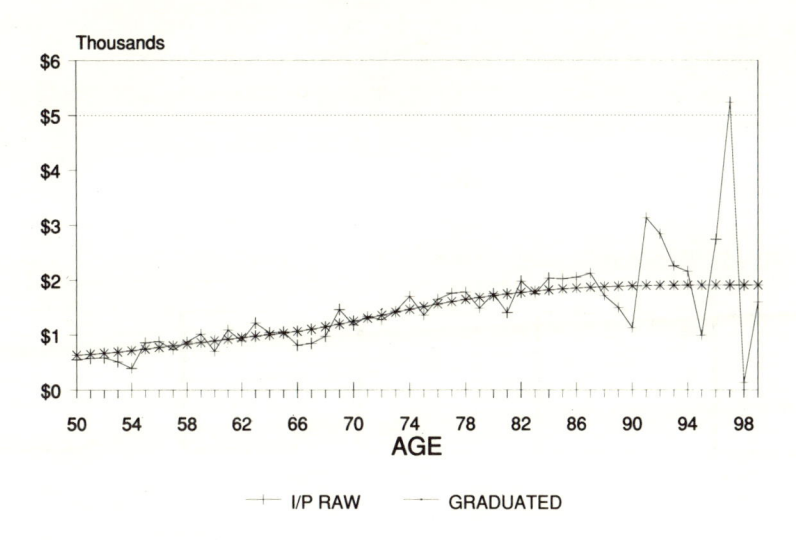

Male and Female Combined

A number of the participating companies did not have sufficient numbers of retirees and dependents to develop a "reliable" cost at each age and by sex and status. Therefore, the graduated average per capita incurred claims cost of those Field Test companies with sufficient claims data was combined, creating a reasonable claims cost pattern by age, sex, and status. This information was used to assist in the estimate of average per capita costs for companies with insufficient claims data. However, the company's own claims experience, even if somewhat limited, was taken into account in establishing average per capita costs.

Trending Forward to 1988

Because January 1, 1988 was assumed to be the date the ED was adopted, it was necessary to adjust or bring forward the experience period information (generally 1986) to 1988. Generally, the following steps were taken:

- 1986 average per capita eligible charges were trended forward on a service sector basis;

- 1986 average per capita deductibles were considered to be representative of 1988 levels;

- 1986 average per capita amounts were expressed as a percentage of 1986 average per capita eligible charges, and that percentage was considered representative of 1988 levels; and

- adjustments were made for any plan design changes that had been implemented by the company during 1986 or 1987 that affected their cost. For example, increased deductibles or coinsurance was considered when bringing costs forward to 1988.

Figure 4.5 illustrates this methodology.

FIGURE 4.5 Trending Forward to 1988

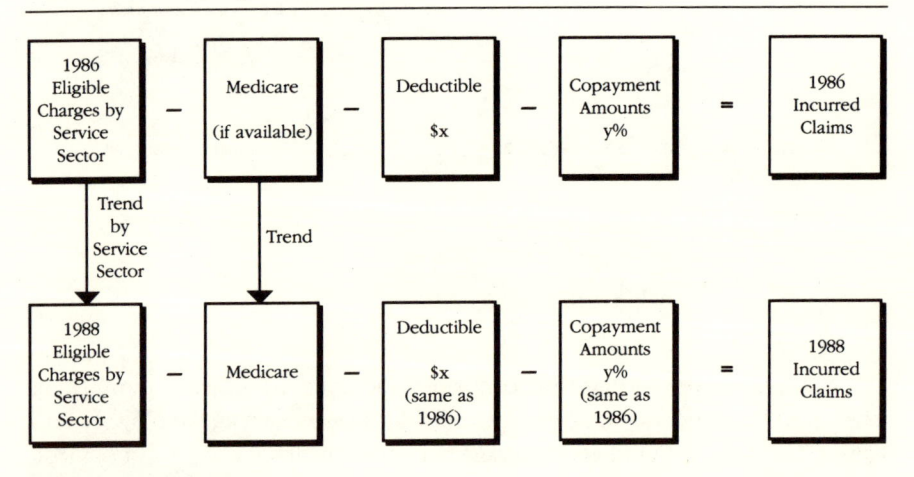

1986 Eligible Charges by Service Sector	−	Medicare (if available)	−	Deductible $x	−	Copayment Amounts y%	=	1986 Incurred Claims
Trend by Service Sector		Trend						
1988 Eligible Charges by Service Sector	−	Medicare	−	Deductible $x (same as 1986)	−	Copayment Amounts y% (same as 1986)	=	1988 Incurred Claims

HMO Information

Almost all of the Field Test companies' HMOs were community rated (i.e., the HMO premiums are based on experience within the region covered by the HMO), and individual or employer-specific claims experience was not available. In addition, HMO participation for those companies offering this option to their retiree group was generally very low, sometimes less than 2 percent. Also, when HMO premium rates were higher than indemnity rates, the retiree was generally required to pay the excess contribution. Therefore, for most of the Field Test companies, retiree HMO participants were assumed to have the same average per capita costs as a retiree of the same age and sex in the companies' comparable indemnity arrangement. Alternatively, annual per capita HMO premiums were used for 65 and over and under 65. For some companies, it was necessary to use 1987 premiums and trend them forward to 1988.

Data Problems and Measurement Issues

As discussed earlier in this chapter, the Field Test began with the collection and analysis of detailed medical claims, demographic, and plan information from the participating companies. In this phase of the study, numerous problems were encountered with the availability and quality of the requested information. These problems required the use of additional assumptions where data was missing or of questionable value.

This section discusses some of the common data problems encountered and addresses the measurement issues associated with the lack of certain data elements.

Examining the Current Benefit Programs

To estimate obligations and expense under the ED it is necessary to clearly understand the terms of the plan provided to retirees. It is, of course, very important to have a thorough understanding of each plan provision that affects cost and the group of employees, retirees, and beneficiaries covered by each plan. Understanding the current coverage was difficult for a number of Field Test companies.

- □ SPDs were frequently out-of-date and had been supplemented by internal memoranda on how the plan was administered. For example, one company's plan document indicated that claim payments were integrated with Medicare using the carve-out method (the least expensive for the employer). In practice, the plan administrator was using the exclusion method to integrate payments with Medicare. As discussed in chapter 9, this has an impact on the magnitude of obligation and expense.

- How the plan was to be administered (e.g., how claims payments were to be integrated with Medicare) was occasionally left to word-of-mouth. Therefore, it was generally necessary and often difficult to locate the appropriate person in each company to confirm how the plan worked in operation. At times it was necessary to contact the insurer or administrator.

Demographic Information

For purposes of a retiree health valuation, it is critical to be able to identify the current retiree group (retirees and their dependents) so that average per capita costs can be developed. Numerous problems were encountered in gathering this detailed information on the relevant retirees and their dependents. Many of the problems discussed below were common for most of the Field Test companies.

- Limited or nonexistent information on spouses and children of retirees was common. Frequently, company eligibility files are maintained based on the retiree's Social Security number, and the existence of dependents as well as detailed information on them is not known (e.g., number and age).

- A number of companies had lump-sum cash-out options in their pension plans. While it was no longer necessary to maintain records for these individuals in the pension eligibility files, many of them were still entitled to retiree health benefits and claims for these individuals appeared in the claims information received.

- Several of the Field Test companies did not maintain historic eligibility information, making it difficult to accurately determine the retirement date or date of death. In addition, some companies did not maintain records of date of birth or date of hire for some retiree groups.

- A number of the companies' eligibility files did not indicate the plan option that a retiree was covered under (e.g., HMO, PPO, or different levels of benefits offered). Since this can affect average per capita costs, it was often necessary to use the claims information to appropriately assign claims to individuals.

- Disabled individuals were frequently not distinguished from early retirees. Disabled individuals may have different health claims experience and mortality rates, which may distort cost estimates if the claims experience for these individuals cannot be analyzed separately.

Observation: Under the ED, disabled individuals on disability retirement would be included in the current retiree population for valuation purposes. In addition, disabled employees who are not yet formally retired would under certain circumstances also be considered to be on disability retirement. For purposes of the Field Test, the terms and intent of the plan determined whether the disabled individuals were treated as currently retired employees.

Medical Claims Information

In the past, employers, insurance carriers, or third-party administrators (TPAs) have generally focused on compiling and storing only the information directly affecting the payment of claims. Therefore, during the data gathering phase of the Field Test, some of the information that would have been helpful in developing average per capita costs for the retiree group was not easily accessible or available from the insurance carrier or the plan administrator.

- One of the most difficult issues encountered in assigning claims to individuals was the lack of uniformity in insurance carrier and TPA administration systems. Different claims administrators code similar information in different ways. It was therefore necessary to understand these different administration systems and to recognize particular "quirks." For example, one claims administration system did not allow for birth dates prior to the year 1900. It appeared, when analyzing 1986 medical claims, as if the particular company utilizing this TPA had many 86-year-olds incurring excessive claims and no claims for older retirees and dependents.

- When an employee or retiree goes to the doctor and incurs a medical expense, there is a lag between when a service is provided and when the related claim is processed for payment. This can be a problem for two reasons:

    —claims incurred during the measurement period may not be processed for payment during the time the data is collected, thereby requiring estimates of these unpaid claims to avoid inappropriately reducing average per capita costs; and

    —claims that were incurred when an individual was an active employee are sometimes not processed until they are retired, thus inappropriately increasing average per capita costs for the retiree group if the status when the claim was incurred is not recognized.

    For purposes of the Field Test, these problems were generally resolved by examining claims paid for an additional six to twelve months after the measurement period and checking the date the service was provided. Also, the status change date (the date the employee became a retiree) was checked against the date medical services were rendered.

- For many of the Field Test companies, there were some claims labeled "retiree" that did not match any individual on the company eligibility files. The claims amounts associated with these "no-match" claims ranged from less than 1 percent of costs to a significant portion of the retiree health care costs. This was caused by a number of different problems such as incomplete historic eligibility files or claims labeled retiree that should have been assigned to an active individual.

- Information as to business unit, salary versus hourly status, or plan type is sometimes not maintained by the claims processors once the claim is paid. This may make it difficult to assign costs to particular employee groups based solely on information provided by the claims processors.

- In addition, some insurance carriers or TPAs do not generally make available information on total eligible charges. Rather, only information on paid claims is available. Coinsurance and other amounts (such as COB and Medicare payments) were frequently not available, creating a number of measurement problems.

- Nearly all of the participating companies provide prescription drug benefits. When administered by an insurance carrier, the usual types of problems (e.g., assigning claims to an individual) occurred. When mail order drug programs were utilized, the problems were exacerbated because a record of claims by individual was not captured. Only "bulk claims" (all claims paid in a certain period) were available in aggregate. A number of the Field Test companies were unable to accurately identify their retirees' claims experience since in many cases, retiree claims were not separated from active employee claims.

Reconciliation to Pay-as-you-go Costs

Under SFAS No. 81, *Disclosure of Postretirement Health Care and Life Insurance Benefits,* companies are currently required to disclose in a footnote to their financial statements, the annual amount charged to expense for their retiree health plans. For companies using pay-as-you-go accounting, this amount is generally based on a summary of paid claims provided by an insurance carrier or TPA. As part of the Field Test, an estimate of benefit payments incurred during 1988 was developed for each of the Field Test companies. A difference often existed between the amount charged to expense and disclosed in the 1988 financial statements and the Field Test estimate of benefit payments. There are a number of reasons for the difference between the reported expense for the Field Test companies and expected incurred benefit payments developed in the Field Test including the following:

- The incurred benefit payments for 1988 developed for the Field Test were estimated, based on actual incurred claims (generally 1986) projected to 1988. The companies' reported expense and disclosure, on the other hand, was generally based on actual claims paid during 1988, usually with an adjustment for lags in claim payments.

- Alternatively, companies used 1987 paid claims information to develop their 1988 pay-as-you-go expense and disclosure amount and estimated an increase in claims paid for the one-year period. This estimate was sometimes based on average paid claims of actives and retirees combined. In projecting 1988 claims based on 1987 data, an adjustment for the impact of different costs and changes in the population distribution under and over age 65 were frequently not included.

- Others computed the paid claim disclosure amounts using average per capita costs for actives and retirees combined multiplied by the number of retirees. The estimates of number of retirees and dependents used by the companies or their insurance carriers may have differed from the estimates used in the Field Test. For example, it is not uncommon in developing the paid claim amount to look at the number of participants at a given point in time, rather than calculating the number of retirees and dependents for the entire period as was done in the Field Test.

Aside from these differences, it is expected that, as with most estimates, there will be a difference between the expected costs and the costs actually incurred. When an actuarial valuation is performed as of January 1 and an assumption is made as to per capita costs, the actual benefit payments for that year will not be known until sometime after the close of the year. The valuation should be completed well before that time. The availability of better information and refinement of the estimation process may reduce the disparity between actual and expected costs.

Conclusion

The data collection and analysis phase of the Field Test was unquestionably the most difficult and time-consuming aspect of the project. However, given the purposes of the study, the detailed methodology was valuable because it provided important information to the companies regarding their underlying costs—where the significant costs for their retiree health program lie. (Chapter 10 provides additional information relating to plan design and the need for data.) Moreover, the Field Test highlighted the practical problems that may be encountered in trying to obtain complete detailed health claims and demographic data.

It is important to note, however, that under the ED, the detailed claims analysis methodology that was developed for the Field Test may not be required for accounting purposes. Retiree health valuations can be performed based on less detailed information; for example, without detailed costs at every age. Each company measuring its obligation and expense under the ED should determine the most appropriate approach given its circumstances and objectives.

Since the Field Test began, many companies and some of their carriers and TPAs have recognized the need for more detailed eligibility and claims information than had traditionally been necessary. However, many companies will still find the estimation of average per capita costs for the retiree group to be a difficult task. As previously discussed, solutions to most of the data problems were found whether by making practical assumptions or looking elsewhere for missing data elements. Companies will find it worthwhile to begin to evaluate the quality and extent of available demographic and medical claims data now so that steps can be taken to assure that necessary information is more readily accessible when it is needed. Accordingly, many companies are considering the following steps.

- ☐ If necessary, upgrade the human resource information system to improve the quality of demographic information, keeping track of status, business unit, plan, and dependent information for each covered employee or retiree. It may be appropriate to introduce more centralized or automated data bases.

- ☐ If not now available, request the insurance carrier or TPA to include additional fields for their edit checks, such as active/retiree status, dependent information, claims incurred data, as well as date paid. Also, modify and expand data reports to increase the information that is readily available.

- ☐ Conduct claims reviews or audits to assure that claims are properly paid and that meaningful financial controls are in place as well as procedures for capturing the needed information.

The Valuation Methodology

As explained earlier, a January 1, 1988 valuation was performed for each company. The active and retiree group as of January 1, 1988 was projected to estimate who will be eligible to receive benefits each succeeding year (the covered retiree group). This type of population projection is commonly referred to as a closed group projection, since new employees are not anticipated.

Recognizing the company's eligibility provisions under each retiree health plan offered, active employees and laid-off employees expected to return to employment as of the valuation date were projected forward using demographic assumptions as to anticipated employee turnover, mortality, retirement, etc., to determine which of these employees are expected to retire and receive benefits under the plans.

Estimating Future Per Capita Costs and Benefit Payments

The benefit payments expected to be made in future years are based on the components of baseline costs discussed above and the covered retiree group each year. In general, average per capita costs for future years are estimated based on economic assumptions as to future trends in health care costs.

In estimating future average per capita costs, average 1988 per capita costs were projected each year. Under the FASB proposal, estimates of future benefit payments would be based on current plan provisions (i.e., future plan changes would not be anticipated). Therefore, it was necessary to keep retiree deductibles and other plan provisions at their specified levels in projecting future costs. Accordingly, as discussed above, in projecting average per capita costs, a cost trend assumption was generally applied to reflect future increases in eligible charges and Medicare (where applicable), while the retiree deductible amounts and copayment percentages were kept at 1988 levels (unless the plan specified increases in cost-sharing or copayment provisions). This stream of future average per capita costs by age is defined as the "assumed per capita costs" in the ED. In other words, the methodology shown in figure 4.5 was followed for each succeeding year as well as for purposes of the January 1, 1988 valuation.

Total employer payments for each future year were determined by applying to the projected covered retiree group for that year, the corresponding per capita costs by age, sex, status (retiree or dependent), and other appropriate breakdowns. Administrative expenses, and where applicable, projected payments for Medicare Part B premiums and contributions by retirees were also used in determining total employer costs for each company.[2]

Present Value of Obligations

The present value of the retiree health care obligations as of the valuation date was determined by discounting to the valuation date the total benefit payments each year using an assumed discount rate selected by each company. Similarly, retiree contributions were discounted and subtracted from the benefit payments to arrive at a net present value amount. Under the ED, companies must look to rates of return on high-quality, fixed-income investments in determining an appropriate discount rate. For a number of the companies, the obligation and expense was also estimated using a discount rate that was based on a company-specific rate to demonstrate the relative impact of this assumption on the obligation and net periodic cost.

Future Year's Valuations

Additional actuarial valuations were performed for nine years after the assumed date of adoption, 1989 to 1997. For these actuarial valuations, it was necessary to project both the current active and retired population forward to each valuation year and recognize new employees entering the workforce each year (referred to as an open group projection). For purposes of this study, average per capita costs and the current population were projected according to the same actuarial assumptions and methods used for the January 1, 1988 valuation. New employees were added each year so that the active population would remain stable, or increased or decreased a certain percentage according to each company's expected change in their workforce.

Notes

1. For purposes of summarizing the valuation results of the Field Test in chapter 6, information from all of a company's plans was aggregated.

2. Only expenses associated with outside administrators such as TPAs or insurance carriers, were taken into account. Any internal administrative costs such as overhead or salaries for internal personnel were not considered.

5
The Health Care Cost Trend and Other Assumptions

The ultimate cost of an employer's retiree health program depends on the benefits provided, the number of individuals utilizing the benefits, and the cost of the health services when they are received. For this reason, obligations cannot be estimated with the same degree of precision as for pension plans, under which benefits are typically determined by a plan formula and are expressed in dollars. Retiree health benefits, on the other hand, are generally not expressed in dollars, and the type, frequency, duration, and cost of future coverage may vary substantially for each covered retiree and dependent. Actuarial assumptions concerning future events are used to make an estimate of future benefit payments and their present value.

Under the ED, the principal actuarial assumptions that would be used to measure obligations and expense include health care cost trend rates, discount rates, the amount and timing of future benefit payments, and the probability of payment. Each significant assumption would reflect the "best estimate" solely with respect to that individual assumption (an explicit approach).

In the Field Test, each company was asked to select its own assumptions based on the guidance provided by the FASB in the ED, taking into consideration its particular facts and circumstances. This chapter briefly describes demographic and other assumptions and provides a summary of research done on the health care cost trend. The key assumptions chosen by the companies are shown in chapter 6. (The assumptions relating to the estimate of average per capita costs are discussed in chapter 4.)

Demographic Assumptions

Many of the demographic assumptions needed for a retiree health plan valuation are comparable to those used in pension plan valuations (anticipated employee turnover, mortality, retirement age, marital status, etc.). However, certain assumptions are unique to measuring retiree health care costs (such as the type of health care delivery system). The same demographic assumptions used in valuing an employer's pension obligation will generally be used in projecting retiree health care obligations for the same covered group of participants. However, the dollar impact of the same assumption on an employer's obligation and expense under each of the two plans will differ because plan benefits and the circumstances under which they are paid differ. These assumptions tend to be more important in measuring retiree health care benefit obligations than in measuring pension obligations. For example:

- The estimate of the number of employees retiring early and their age at retirement can affect retiree health care costs significantly since Medicare generally does not become the primary payer until the retiree reaches age 65. In addition, there is generally no reduced health benefit for early retirement—the full benefit is immediately payable and remains payable over a longer period of time.

- Many retiree health plans provide coverage for the lives of spouses of retirees. As a result, assumptions must be made as to the number of employees who are expected to be married at and during retirement. An assumption must also be made concerning the ages of the spouses. Under a pension plan, a spousal benefit is payable only after the death of a retiree and is generally payable as a percentage of the retiree's pension (not to exceed 100 percent). Further, spousal pension benefits are often financed, at least in part, by a reduction in the retiree's pension. Spousal retiree health benefits, on the other hand, often cost an employer more than health benefits for the retiree—currently most retirees are male and their spouses are female. (Females have a longer life expectancy causing benefits to be paid over a longer period of time than males.) This makes the marital status assumption of particular importance when valuing retiree health benefits.

□ An assumption may also need to be made for the number of nonspouse dependents covered by retiree health plans. While there is generally no similar assumption needed for pension plans, under some situations nonspouse dependent health care coverage can be costly.

For these reasons, the Field Test companies were encouraged to carefully review each significant assumption selected for valuing their retiree health care benefit programs.

Economic Assumptions

The Health Care Cost Trend

The health care cost trend assumption is applied to per capita costs every year to estimate a company's stream of future costs. Under the ED, this is referred to as assumed per capita costs. For purposes of the Field Test, the health care cost trend was generally applied to eligible charges (usually net of Medicare) for each year. (See chapter 4 for additional information.)

Under the ED, in determining the health care cost trend assumption, estimates of health care inflation, changes in health care utilization or delivery patterns, technological advances, and changes in the health status of plan participants would be considered. Further, the ED states that different services, such as hospital care and dental services, may require different health care trend rates; and that it is appropriate to reflect in that assumption that these rates may change over time.

For accounting purposes, the health care cost trend rate assumption is unique to the measurement of retiree health care benefits. Uncertainty surrounding the likely course of future economic events complicates estimating trend rates for a period that may exceed 70 years. Because of the importance of this assumption in estimating obligations and expense, and because there is little readily available information for companies to refer to when attempting to choose reasonable assumptions, extensive economic research was performed to provide guidance to the Field Test companies so they could select trend rates appropriate for their situation. Estimates of obligations and expense were also performed for the Field Test companies utilizing alternative trend rates.

Observation: Predicting the health care cost trend over an extended period of time is a difficult challenge and one that leaves open many important questions. The research presented in this chapter was conducted in an effort to comply with the requirements in the ED while providing companies information that would place them in a better position to evaluate the specific criteria contained in the ED. In this regard, a number of the Field Test companies believe that either a 0 percent trend assumption, an assumption based on general inflation, or a trend assumption based solely on health care price inflation would provide more meaningful and consistent financial information.

The following discussion summarizes the economic research performed for the Field Test.

Research on Health Care Economic Trends and Assumptions

Introduction

Apart from the number and demographic mix of its retirees and their dependents, a company's spending for retiree health benefits depends partly on price levels, utilization rates, intensity of services delivered, and Medicare policies. From an historical perspective, continuation of past trends will cause employers to spend significantly larger sums for retiree health benefits. From a national perspective, continuation will cause health services to absorb a mounting proportion of Gross National Product (GNP).

This section explains a method to estimate the health care economic trend factors that would be used to project retiree health benefit costs under the ED. This method was developed after an extensive review of the economic literature addressing future health care costs. The section explains the research conducted, identifies the six health service categories used in the Field Test for projection purposes, defines the components of the economic trend factors, and analyzes historical factors contributing to health expenditure growth. Subsequently, the projected health care trend factors are presented and discussed.

Each Field Test company was presented with a summary of this research. The purpose was to provide them with guidance in selecting appropriate health care cost trend rates as required under the ED.

Literature Survey

Professional literature published during the last decade was surveyed to identify economic models that project health expenditures. The research focused on stand-alone health care models and macroeconomic models with health care as a separate component. The findings suggest that the former models are currently more appropriate for projecting retiree health benefits. Four stand-alone models were investigated in detail:

- ☐ University of Southern California Microeconomic Simulation Model;
- ☐ National Institute of Aging Macroeconomic Demographic Model;

- Medicare Model; and
- Health Care Financing Administration (HCFA) Projection Model.

The assessment of each model's structure, properties, estimation techniques, and data requirements led to the adoption of a modified version of the last two models. First, much of the microeconomic and macroeconomic information needed to tailor the other two models to employers is not available.

Second, substantial doubt prevails about whether the greater computational sophistication and theoretical elegance of the other two models would improve forecasting accuracy enough to justify the additional cost, if at all. Third, the complexity of the other two models could limit their acceptability.

Health Service Categories

Figure 5.1 depicts in general terms the computational process to project an employer's retiree health costs in a specific year. For a category of service and demographic class, an employer's current population (the number of persons in the class) is multiplied by per capita cost. The product is then increased by the economic trend factor for each service.

FIGURE 5.1

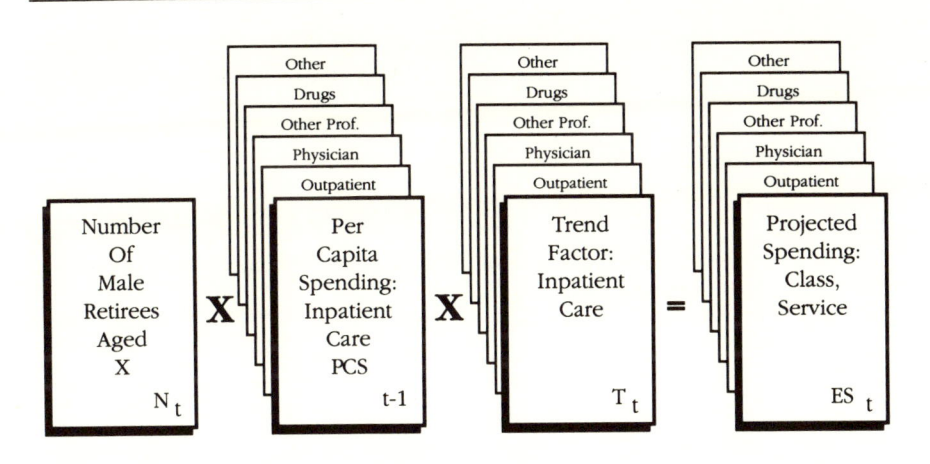

Number Of Male Retirees Aged X N_t X Per Capita Spending: Inpatient Care PCS $t-1$ X Trend Factor: Inpatient Care T_t = Projected Spending: Class, Service ES_t

(categories: Outpatient, Physician, Other Prof., Drugs, Other)

Health service categories can be organized in numerous ways. For example, services can be clustered into diagnostic and procedural codes. Services for different groups of providers can be combined. Institutional services can be split from noninstitutional services; general acute inpatient care from long-term or specialty care. Medicare covered services can be separated from noncovered services.

After assessing various options, the following six service categories were established: (1) inpatient hospital care, (2) outpatient hospital care, (3) physician services and independent laboratories, (4) drugs and medical sundries, (5) other professional services, and (6) all other items. In general, these categories resemble the National Health Accounts, with the major exception that hospital care is separated into inpatient and outpatient components. The federal government uses the National Health Accounts, or service categories, to tabulate health expenditures nationwide. In addition, the service categories used for the Field Test resemble the categories that the models used to project health expenditures.

Economic Trend Factor

Under the ED, the health care trend factor is generally based on the projected rate of change in an employer's per capita eligible charges for reasons other than a change in demographic mix or a change in the employer's retiree health plan. Defined this way, the trend factor would measure expected changes in health care prices, utilization, and service intensity. (Under the guidance in the ED, the trend would be applied to gross eligible charges before Medicare, but as discussed in chapter 4, this data was generally not available.)

- Health Care Prices—This component is intended to measure nationwide increases in the unit price of a given health service or commodity. For each service, this component is split into an economy-wide measure of general inflation, and the excess of health inflation over the economy-wide rate.

- Utilization Rate—This component addresses changes in the number (not mix) of services, as measured by patient days, discharges, visits, procedures, or other units of service. The projections are based on past utilization experiences of the national population and Medicare beneficiaries.

- Service Intensity—This component deals with changes in the mix or content of specific units of service, such as hospital days, physician visits, and prescriptions. Change in service intensity may reinforce or counter changes in utilization. For example, in the case of inpatient hospital care, the mix of inpatient days may change or the amount of care rendered during a typical day may change due to a greater number of different and more sophisticated tests being performed.

- Medicare Policies—As primary payer for a major portion of the health services that retirees receive, Medicare coverage and reimbursement policies have a significant bearing on an employer's retiree health care obligations.

The magnitude depends on how an employer's retiree plan coordinates with Medicare. For purposes of the ED, however, current Medicare law is assumed not to change in the future.

An employer's future per capita health costs also will depend on technological developments and regulatory requirements. In the past, changes in both of these variables have tended to increase costs. The cost consequences of these changes were not factored separately into the health care trend factor. Rather, they are embedded in the projections for health care inflation, utilization, and service intensity.

Sensitivity analysis. Any attempt to estimate a trend factor will, of course, require judgment regarding complex future events. Individuals may interpret historical information differently or have divergent views about the future. Moreover, long-term economic trends cannot be predicted with a high degree of confidence. Trend factors were therefore prepared under three scenarios—optimistic, best estimate, and pessimistic—to gauge their sensitivity to varying assumptions.

Historical growth. Table 5.1 shows national average annual rates of change for factors affecting the growth in the national spending for several health services dating back to 1965. The figures show the following.

- As shown by comparing the "inflation" column to the "total change" column, for almost every time interval, medical inflation (health care prices) has accounted for over one-half of the expenditure growth, except for outpatient hospital care and drugs. Increases in health care prices usually have outpaced national inflation rates. The excess amount has fluctuated considerably over time. For drugs and medical sundries, the excess amount has ranged from −4.04 percent between 1970 and 1975 to 3.81 percent in 1986.

- Service intensity has changed considerably but erratically over time. Hospital care has registered the largest gains. Between 1980 and 1985, the service intensity of inpatient and outpatient care each increased over 7.6 percent a year, not counting changes related to demographic mix. In contrast, service intensity for drugs and medical supplies appears to have declined about 1.5 percent a year since 1980.

- Utilization of outpatient hospital services has increased significantly faster than utilization of all the other medical services. Utilization of the other services frequently has risen less than 1 percent a year. And, in the case of inpatient hospital care, utilization has declined about 5 percent a year since

TABLE 5.1 Average Annual Change in Factors Contributing to Increases in Spending for Selected Health Services, 1965-1986

Service and year	Factors related to demographic mix - Utilization	Factors related to demographic mix - Intensity	Factors other than demographic mix - Utilization	Factors other than demographic mix - Intensity	Inflation National	Inflation Excess	Population growth	Total change
Inpatient hospital care								
1965-1970	0.45%	0.01%	1.43%	6.54%	4.48%	1.92%	1.05%	16.79%
1970-1975	0.62	(0.05)	(0.56)	4.14	7.13	0.54	0.88	13.18
1975-1980	0.69	(0.06)	0.17	4.60	7.63	1.05	0.92	15.75
1980-1985	0.66	(0.09)	(5.03)	7.61	5.41	0.90	0.99	10.40
1985-1986	0.68	(0.10)	(3.00)	4.65	2.71	0.28	0.93	6.15
Outpatient hospital care								
1965-1970	(0.01%)	0.12%	7.29%	3.03%	4.48%	1.92%	1.05%	19.05%
1970-1975	0.04	0.13	6.14	2.63	7.13	0.54	0.88	18.58
1975-1980	0.06	0.11	1.48	6.29	7.63	1.05	0.92	18.63
1980-1985	0.07	0.06	1.18	7.73	5.41	0.90	0.99	17.22
1985-1986	0.05	0.06	7.28	4.97	2.71	0.28	0.93	17.19
Physician services								
1965-1970	0.07%	0.14%	0.82%	2.13%	4.48%	1.98%	1.05%	11.10%
1970-1975	0.18	0.19	1.45	1.70	7.13	(0.19)	0.88	11.70
1975-1980	0.26	0.17	(0.09)	2.13	7.63	1.92	0.92	13.44
1980-1985	0.24	0.09	0.24	1.97	5.41	2.63	0.99	12.05
1985-1986	0.22	0.10	0.01	2.34	2.71	4.37	0.93	11.10
Dental services								
1965-1970	0.24%	0.10%	(1.05%)	5.13%	4.48%	0.79%	1.05%	11.08%
1970-1975	0.15	0.13	1.29	2.50	7.13	(0.79)	0.88	11.64
1975-1980	0.01	0.11	0.50	3.16	7.63	0.52	0.92	13.35
1980-1985	(0.10)	0.05	2.41	0.54	5.41	2.18	0.99	11.93
1985-1986	(0.07)	0.05	0.97	1.78	2.71	2.82	0.93	9.50
Drugs and medical sundries								
1965-1970	0.17%	0.05%	0.82%[a]	6.12%[b]	4.48	(3.66%)	1.05%	9.07%
1970-1975	0.28	0.06	1.45	2.64	7.13	(4.04)	0.88	8.35
1975-1980	0.36	0.05	(0.09)	0.86	7.63	(0.42)	0.92	9.45
1980-1985	0.34	0.03	0.24	(1.55)	5.41	3.24	0.99	8.87
1985-1986	0.36	0.04	0.01	(1.42)	2.71	3.81	0.93	6.50

[a] The numbers in this column are set at the rates for physician services because the utilization of physician visits and prescribed drugs have been found to be highly correlated.

[b] The numbers in this column must be viewed with exceptional caution due to data constraints.

Source: Health Care Financing Administration.

1980. The substantial drop in admissions and average lengths of stay may stem partly from the implementation of Medicare's prospective payment system in 1983 and the subsequent growth in prepaid and managed health plans.

- Changes in demographic mix (age and gender) have had a relatively nominal effect on total spending. Most of the annual changes are below 0.40 percent; only four (all for inpatient hospital care) exceed 0.50 percent.

Projected growth. Tables 5.2 and 5.3 show service-specific economic trend factors for 1988 to 2070 based on the economic research previously discussed. These factors are average annual rates of projected increase, typically spanning five-year intervals. The trend factors in table 5.2 reflect compounded changes in projected per capita utilization and service intensity due to factors other than changes in demographic mix. The trend factors in table 5.3 reflect the rates in table 5.2 plus projected health care inflation rates. General economy-wide inflation was assumed to increase 4.5 percent a year between 1988 and 2070. (To put this increase in perspective, the GNP deflator rose 4.6 percent a year between 1980 and 1987; 3.2 percent between 1982 and 1987; 4.8 percent for the 30 years ending in 1987.) The excess of medical inflation over economy-wide inflation is assumed to vary by service and to decrease over time.

As seen in table 5.3, health care economic trend factors were projected under three scenarios. Using the criteria required in the ED, the alternative sets of assumptions comprise a range over which employer spending for retiree health benefits reasonably might be expected to increase between 1988 and 2070. Typically, until 2020 the trend factors in Scenario B ("best estimate") are about six-tenths of a percentage point higher than Scenario A ("optimistic"); likewise for Scenario C ("pessimistic") relative to Scenario B. After 2020, the differences between the scenarios narrow considerably. Trend factors lower than those in Scenario A were not prepared because Scenario A was deemed to be conservative relative to historical experience.

Scenario B represents a best estimate in the context of the proposed requirements in the ED. Scenario A is deemed low because Americans have repeatedly demonstrated a willingness to spend more for additional health services than the increase in per capita real GNP. Also, expected declines in the rate of increase in service intensity appear optimistic, particularly through the year 2000. Scenario C seems high because its growth rates approximate the past too closely, a time when financial arrangements and societal attitudes were more supportive of expenditure growth.

TABLE 5.2 Average Annual Change in Projected Economic Trend Factors Exclusive of Medical Inflation, by Type of Service and Scenario, 1988-2070 (Excludes expenditure growth due to changes in the number and demographic mix of retirees and dependents)

Scenario and year	Inpatient hospital care	Outpatient hospital care	Physician services	Drugs and medical sundries	Other professional services	All other services
Scenario A						
1988-1990	1.5%	5.5%	1.8%	1.8%	2.3%	1.7%
1990-1995	1.5	4.0	1.5	1.4	1.9	1.5
1995-2000	1.4	3.0	1.4	1.0	1.7	1.4
2000-2005	1.3	2.5	1.3	0.8	1.5	1.3
2005-2010	1.2	2.0	1.3	0.5	1.4	1.3
2010-2015	1.1	1.5	1.2	0.3	1.2	1.2
2015-2020	1.0	1.5	1.1	0.3	1.1	1.1
2020-2050	1.0	1.3	0.9	0.3	1.1	1.0
2050-2070	1.0	1.1	0.9	0.3	1.1	1.0
Scenario B						
1988-1990	1.8%	6.0%	2.1%	2.1%	2.6%	2.0%
1990-1995	1.8	4.5	1.8	1.7	2.2	1.8
1995-2000	1.7	3.5	1.7	1.3	2.0	1.7
2000-2005	1.6	3.0	1.6	1.1	1.8	1.6
2005-2010	1.5	2.5	1.6	0.8	1.7	1.6
2010-2015	1.4	2.0	1.5	0.6	1.5	1.5
2015-2020	1.3	2.0	1.4	0.6	1.4	1.4
2020-2050	1.2	1.3	1.2	0.6	1.3	1.2
2050-2070	1.0	1.2	1.0	0.6	0.9	1.0
Scenario C						
1988-1990	2.1%	6.5%	2.4%	2.4%	2.9%	2.3%
1990-1995	2.1	5.0	2.1	2.0	2.5	2.1
1995-2000	2.0	4.0	2.0	1.6	2.3	2.0
2000-2005	1.9	3.5	1.9	1.4	2.1	1.9
2005-2010	1.8	3.0	1.9	1.1	2.0	1.9
2010-2015	1.7	2.5	1.8	0.9	1.8	1.8
2015-2020	1.6	2.5	1.7	0.9	1.7	1.7
2020-2050	1.4	1.5	1.3	0.9	1.4	1.4
2050-2070	1.1	1.2	1.1	0.9	1.0	1.1

Source: Coopers & Lybrand

TABLE 5.3 Average Annual Change in Projected Economic Trend Factors Inclusive of Medical Inflation, by Type of Service and Scenario, 1988-2070 (Excludes expenditure growth due to changes in the number and demographic mix of retirees and dependents)

Scenario and year	Inpatient hospital care	Outpatient hospital care	Physician services	Drugs and medical sundries	Other professional services	All other services
Scenario A						
1988-1990	7.2%	11.5%	9.0%	8.8%	8.5%	8.1%
1990-1995	7.0	9.7	8.0	7.8	7.8	7.5
1995-2000	6.7	8.4	7.6	6.9	7.3	7.1
2000-2005	6.6	7.9	7.2	6.4	6.8	6.9
2005-2010	6.3	7.1	6.9	5.8	6.5	6.6
2010-2015	6.2	6.6	6.5	5.3	6.1	6.3
2015-2020	5.9	6.4	6.2	5.3	5.8	6.0
2020-2050	5.9	6.2	6.1	5.2	5.7	6.0
2050-2070	5.9	6.0	6.1	5.1	5.7	6.0
Scenario B						
1988-1990	7.8%	12.2%	9.7%	9.5%	9.2%	8.7%
1990-1995	7.6	10.4	8.6	8.4	8.4	8.1
1995-2000	7.2	9.1	8.2	7.6	8.0	7.7
2000-2005	7.1	8.6	7.9	7.0	7.5	7.5
2005-2010	6.8	7.9	7.6	6.4	7.1	7.2
2010-2015	6.7	7.3	7.1	6.0	6.7	6.9
2015-2020	6.4	7.1	6.8	6.0	6.4	6.6
2020-2050	6.2	6.3	6.4	5.5	6.0	6.3
2050-2070	6.0	6.2	6.1	5.2	5.7	6.0
Scenario C						
1988-1990	8.3%	13.0%	10.3%	10.1%	9.8%	9.3%
1990-1995	8.1	11.2	9.3	9.1	9.1	8.7
1995-2000	7.8	9.9	8.8	8.2	8.6	8.3
2000-2005	7.7	9.3	8.5	7.7	8.1	8.1
2005-2010	7.3	8.6	8.2	7.0	7.8	7.8
2010-2015	7.2	8.1	7.8	6.6	7.3	7.5
2015-2020	6.9	7.9	7.4	6.6	7.0	7.2
2020-2050	6.5	6.6	6.6	5.9	6.2	6.6
2050-2070	6.1	6.2	6.3	5.5	5.9	6.2

Source: Coopers & Lybrand

Health Care as a Proportion of GNP

Projections of health expenditures on a national basis typically are accompanied by projections of health expenditures as a proportion of GNP. Projected proportions can be used to screen the plausibility of the underlying economic assumptions. Strong skepticism about the assumptions can be expected whenever a proportion exceeds a certain threshold or is predicted to grow rapidly over a short time. Individuals differ in their perceptions of the maximum proportion of GNP that society would be willing to devote to health care. Some observers place the upward boundary at approximately 20 percent; many challenge 30 percent as a realistic option. Projections above an established threshold are apt to result in the assumptions being revised.

Since Medicare's enactment in 1965, health care has steadily absorbed an increasing share of GNP. In 1987, all personal health care expenditures combined accounted for 9.8 percent of GNP, up from 9.3 percent in 1985 and 5.1 percent in 1965.[1] This rapid growth manifests society's accelerating demand for health care as its income increases. A similar phenomenon, but at lower proportions of GNP, has occurred in other western industrialized nations.

Personal health expenditures will absorb an estimated 13.3 percent of the GNP in year 2000 and 18.1 percent in 2020 if the projections for Scenario B in table 5.3 materialize nationwide. Table 5.4 also shows personal health care as a percent of GNP for Scenarios A and C. These estimates include amounts for expenditure growth attributable to changes in the demographic mix of the national population.

TABLE 5.4   Personal Health Care Expenditures as a Percentage of GNP

Year	Scenario A	Scenario B	Scenario C
2000	12.3%	13.3%	14.5%
2010	13.7	15.7	18.1
2020	14.9	18.1	22.0

Conclusion

The inherent uncertainty surrounding future economic events vastly complicates efforts to predict employer spending for retiree health benefits, particularly over the long run. This uncertainty complicated the development of projections under different economic scenarios. Together (following the criteria proposed in the ED), these scenarios form a range over which employer spending for retiree health benefits may reasonably be expected to fall during the projection period.

Projected health care economic trend factors were derived from information based on national population trends and Medicare beneficiaries. This information may not be representative of an employer's retiree health benefit claims experience.

Observation: Several Field Test companies thought the projected trend rates were low for 1988 through 2000. Some of the companies had just received large increases in their health insurance premiums. Others were experiencing claims payment increases well above national rates of increase. Accordingly, a number of the companies used higher trend rates in the early years (e.g., one or two percentage points higher) than the best estimate provided in the research. In addition, a few other Field Test companies considered the trends low because they were thinking in terms of their company's net payments rather than eligible charges. Applying the health care cost trend to eligible charges (as was done in the Field Test) results in a higher percentage increase in net payments than the trends shown in the research (for example, due to leveraging of the deductible).

HMO Trend Assumptions

HMO costs were not available on a service-sector basis. In addition, HMO costs may be assumed to rise at a rate, in the aggregate, that differs from costs under an indemnity arrangement. Accordingly, separate HMO trend rates were developed, based on the economic research done for health care cost trends in general. The Field Test companies with a significant number of retirees participating in HMOs were provided with guidance in selecting the HMO trend rates appropriate for their particular circumstances. As discussed in chapter 4, the majority of the Field Test companies had very few retirees covered by HMOs.

The Discount Rate

Under the ED, the discount rate would reflect the rates at which the benefits could be effectively settled. Employers could look to current rates of return on high-quality, fixed-income investments in selecting these rates.

Observation: It is important to note that unlike pensions there are currently very few products on the market whereby a company could effectively settle its obligation for retiree health benefits.

The assumed discount rate tends to counterbalance the effect of the health care cost trend assumption. The higher the discount rate, the lower the present value of projected obligations. The opposite is true for health care cost trend assumptions. In selecting a discount rate, the ED would require that the underlying inflation component be consistent with that used for the health care cost trend.

Each Field Test company selected a discount rate to estimate obligations and expense consistent with the ED requirements. Chapter 6 provides information on the discount rate selected by the Field Test companies.

The ED would require the discount rate to change each year to reflect the current rates at which benefits could be effectively settled. The impact of changing the discount rate would be reflected as an actuarial gain or loss. For purposes of the Field Test, however, gains and losses were not reflected in the estimate of obligations and expense for 1989 and later years.

As part of the Field Test, a number of companies also selected a company-specific rate based on the company's average or marginal interest rate on borrowing, cost of capital or return on equity. Certain Field Test companies and others believe this may be appropriate since, unlike pension obligations, employers generally self-finance these obligations—either by raising additional capital or by diverting retained earnings from other uses.

Sensitivity analyses were performed to demonstrate the effect of using the different discount rates. The results are shown in chapter 6.

Other Assumptions

Employers' retiree health programs vary greatly. As a result, a number of other assumptions may be necessary. Examples of other assumptions made by the Field Test companies follow.

- Companies may need to make an assumption about the number of eligible retirees who will eventually participate in the plan. This assumption is separate from the mortality assumption and takes into account nonparticipation for reasons such as better coverage under a spouse's health plan.

- For some companies, the percentage of future retirees who will enroll in HMOs versus indemnity arrangements must be estimated. This assumption may be particularly important for companies that expect per capita HMO costs to be less than the cost of indemnity arrangements.

- An assumption is generally needed relative to the percentage increase in administrative expenses (out-of-pocket only). This increase may not be the same rate as the general rate of inflation or health care inflation.

Notes

1. These percentages include personal health care only. National health expenditures include personal health care as well as program administration and the cost of insurance, government public health activities, and the research and construction of medical facilities. National health expenditures represented 11.2 percent of GNP in 1987.

6
Valuation Results

The ED's impact on retiree health benefit obligations and expense was analyzed for each Field Test company, with a specific focus on:

- Obligations and expense under the ED for the year of adoption and future years;
- Sensitivity of obligations and expense to alternate health care cost trend and discount rate assumptions;
- Impact of alternative approaches to various provisions contained in the ED on obligations and expense; and
- Analysis of accrued and minimum liability provisions.

The results presented in this chapter were based on the actuarial valuations performed for each company in the Field Test (assuming adoption of the proposed statement for 1988) using assumptions selected by each company and the actuarial methods described in chapter 4. In presenting Field Test results, the "best estimate" health care cost trend rates and discount rate assumptions selected by the companies (based on the guidance in the ED) were used, except in the analysis of sensitivity to changes in assumptions. In years following the adoption of the proposed statement, the Field Test valuations assumed that actual experience would follow the actuarial assumptions used in the initial valuation (i.e., no gains or losses). Further, it was assumed that there were no plan amendments.

Because most retiree health plans are currently unfunded and accounted for on a pay-as-you-go basis, the Field Test results presented in this chapter do not consider any plan assets or accrued liabilities on the companies' balance sheets at the date of transition. In addition, special accounting provisions of certain industries (e.g., utilities, insurance, brokerage) were not considered in the Field Test. Results for an individual company may represent a composite of the results for two or more plans.

Hypothetical Examples and Field Test Results

In order for the companies participating in the Field Test to remain anonymous, specific company obligations and expense amounts have not been presented. Instead, the computed results for two realistic hypothetical companies are presented. While these two companies were not actual participants in the Field Test, their demographics and costs are similar to those of several Field Test companies. Calculated dollar amounts for these companies are discussed initially to enable readers to better understand actual Field Test results, which follow the illustrative results.

Company demographics and the specific benefits offered by a company significantly affect the measurement of retiree health obligations and expense. In particular, the ratio of the number of active employees to the number of retirees is an important factor in understanding the financial impact of applying the ED. For the Field Test, the participating companies were classified according to their ratio of retirees (excluding dependents) to active employees (see chapter 12), as follows:[1]

Classification	Demographic Characteristic	Number of Field Test Companies
Highly Mature	Less than two active employees for every retiree	9
Mature	Two to six active employees for every retiree	13
Immature	More than six active employees for every retiree	4
		26

The hypothetical company labeled "highly mature" has slightly less than two active employees for every retiree. The hypothetical company with more active employees—approximately one retiree for every ten actives—is labeled "immature." All other demographic characteristics (e.g., average age of retirees, dependents and active employees), as well as plan provisions, were identical for both hypothetical companies. Figure 6.1 presents the participant profiles of the two hypothetical companies.

FIGURE 6.1 Plan Participant Profiles — Hypothetical Companies

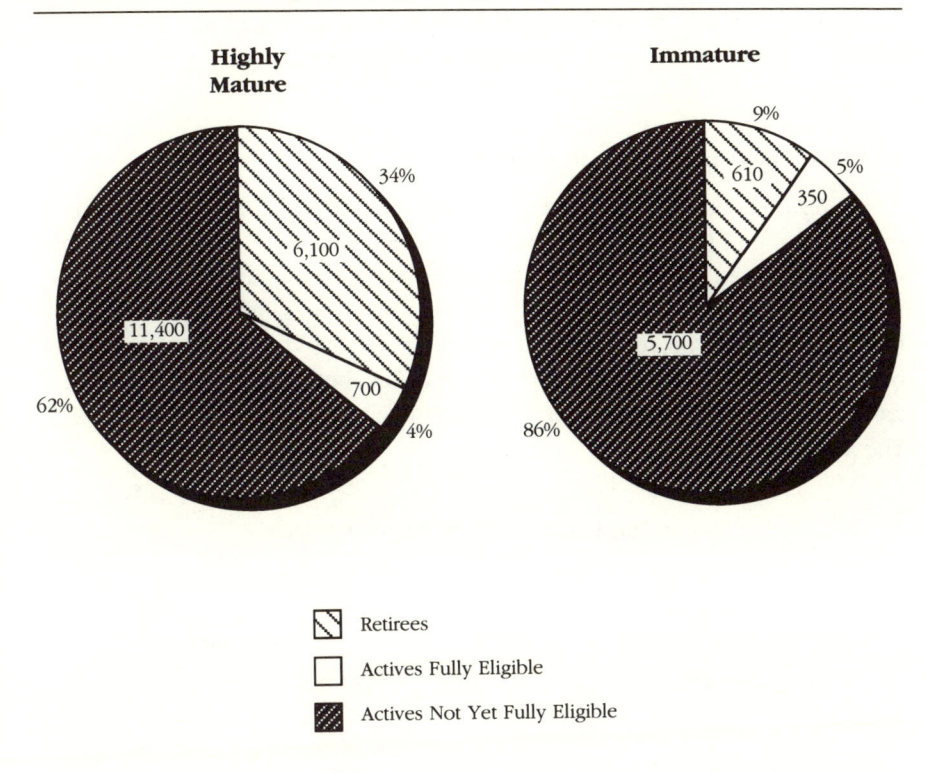

Highly Mature
- 34% — 6,100
- 62% — 11,400
- 4% — 700

Immature
- 9% — 610
- 5% — 350
- 86% — 5,700

Legend:
- Retirees
- Actives Fully Eligible
- Actives Not Yet Fully Eligible

Caution: The obligations and expense amounts for the two hypothetical companies should be used by readers as illustrations of the possible impact of applying accrual accounting. The actual impact on a particular company's financial statements will vary because of a number of factors, including the unique features of its benefit program, its specific demographics, and the assumptions used in the actuarial measurements. Therefore, each company should specifically measure its obligations and expense under the FASB proposal, since the results may vary significantly based on a company's specific facts and circumstances.

Obligations

Retiree health obligations and expense under accrual accounting are determined by the measurement of the actuarial present value of benefits expected to be paid after retirement—the expected postretirement benefit obligation (EPBO). Under the ED, the EPBO is attributed to different periods based on employee service. As discussed more completely in chapter 3, the portion of the EPBO attributed to employee service up to the measurement date is called the accumulated postretirement benefit obligation (APBO). The remainder of the EPBO relates to future service which would be charged to expense in future years as service cost.

Comparing the APBO and EPBO

Figure 6.2 presents the EPBO and the APBO for the hypothetical companies as of the beginning of the year that accrual accounting is adopted. These obligations were determined using the FASB's proposed methodology and guidance on actuarial assumptions. All actuarial assumptions were the same for the two hypothetical companies presented. Measurements were based on the "best estimate" health care cost trend rates developed from the economic research conducted as part of the Field Test (see chapter 5) and a 9¼ percent discount rate assumption. The plans are unfunded.

FIGURE 6.2   Obligations (in Millions) — Hypothetical Companies

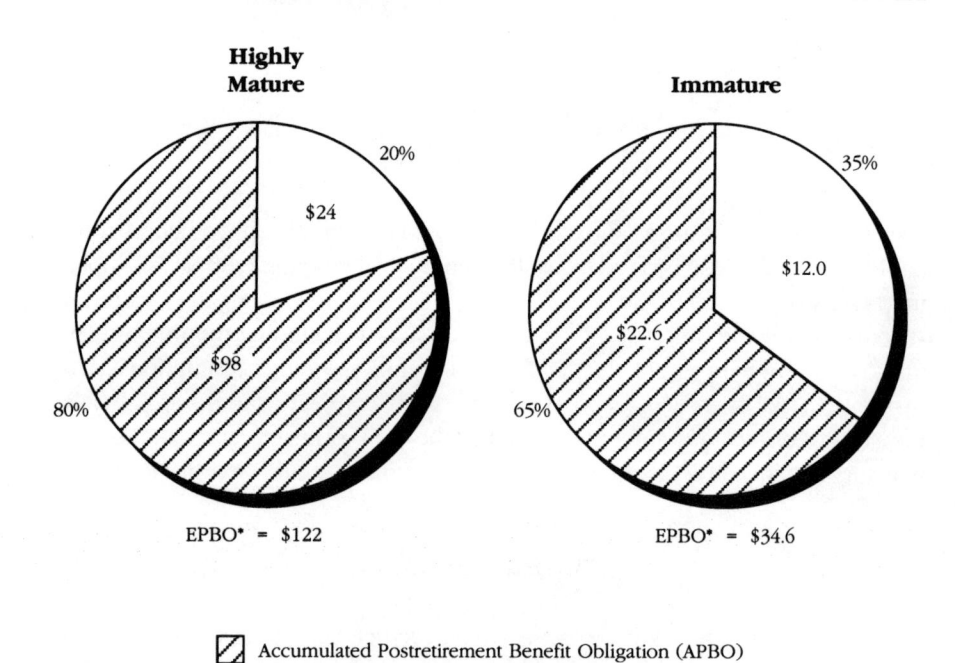

Highly Mature

20%
$24
$98
80%

EPBO* = $122

Immature

35%
$12.0
$22.6
65%

EPBO* = $34.6

▨ Accumulated Postretirement Benefit Obligation (APBO)
☐ Present Value Future Service Costs
• Expected Postretirement Benefit Obligation

Field Test Results

For the highly mature hypothetical company with a large retiree base, 80 percent of the EPBO at the date of adoption relates to past service (the APBO). For all of the highly mature Field Test companies, the APBO comprised over 78 percent of the EPBO. For a few "highly mature" companies with more retirees than active employees, the APBO comprised nearly 90 percent or more of the EPBO.

For the immature hypothetical company, the APBO was 65 percent of the EPBO. Since most Field Test companies tended toward the mature end of the spectrum, few actual Field Test companies exhibited this relationship. All four immature Field Test companies showed a relationship of APBO to EPBO of less than 75 percent, with most less than 67 percent. Table 6.1 presents a summary of results.

TABLE 6.1 APBO as Percentage of EPBO

	Highly Mature	Mature	Immature	Total
Number of companies:				
Less than 60%	0	0	2	2
60—69%	0	1	1	2
70—79%	2	7	1	10
80—89%	5	5	0	10
90% and greater	2	0	0	2
	9	13	4	26

Components of the APBO

The APBO includes obligations relating to three groups of plan participants:

- retirees and their dependents (referred to as "retirees");
- active employees fully eligible for benefits and their assumed dependents (referred to as "eligibles"); and
- active employees not yet fully eligible for benefits and their assumed dependents (referred to as "actives not yet eligible").

86 *Retiree Health Benefits*

FIGURE 6.3 Accumulated Postretirement Benefit Obligation (in Millions) — Hypothetical Companies

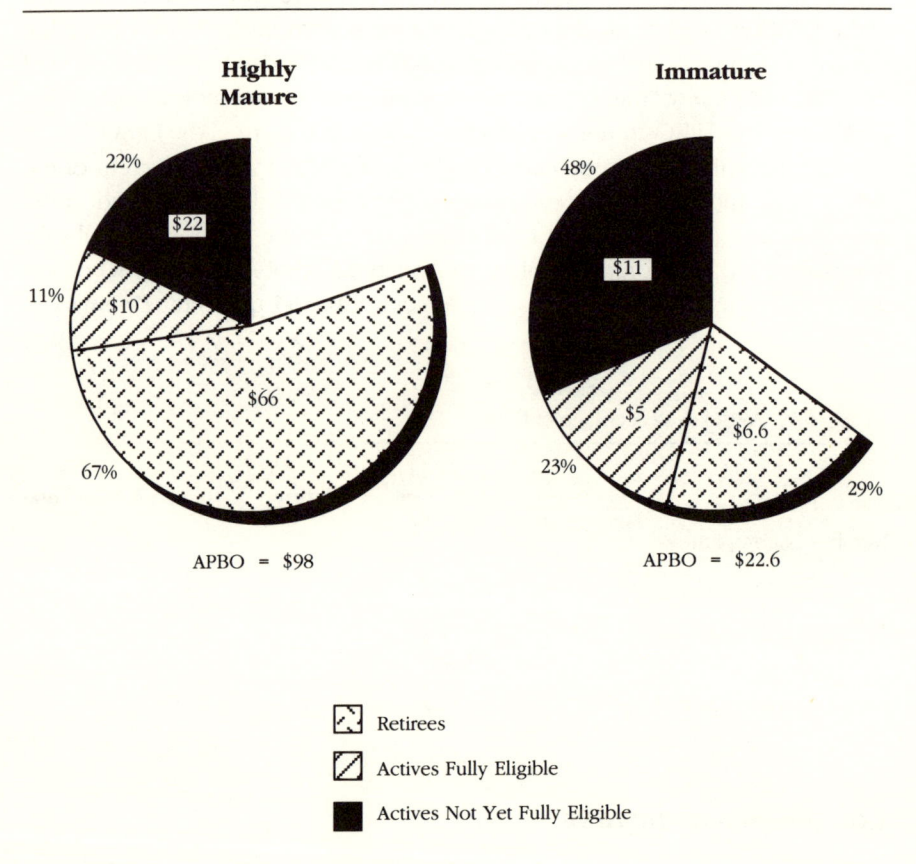

Highly Mature

22% $22
11% $10
67% $66

APBO = $98

Immature

48% $11
23% $5
29% $6.6

APBO = $22.6

- Retirees
- Actives Fully Eligible
- Actives Not Yet Fully Eligible

Field Test Results

Table 6.2 summarizes results regarding the components of the APBO for the Field Test companies at date of assumed adoption of the ED. A number of the Field Test companies exhibited patterns similar to those shown by the hypothetical companies when looking at the breakdown of the APBO by component (i.e., retirees, eligibles, and actives not yet eligible). There were three highly mature cases in which over 72 percent of the APBO related to retirees, and two very immature cases, in which over 30 percent of the APBO related to retirees.

The eligible component of the APBO ranged from 10 to 20 percent for most Field Test companies. Most mature Field Test companies showed over 16 percent of the APBO attributable to the eligible component, and over 30 percent of the APBO attributable to actives not yet eligible. For almost all of the highly mature Field Test companies, the eligible component of the APBO was less than 16 percent and the component of the APBO for active employees not yet eligible was under 30 percent. In addition to the demographic characteristics of the active and retiree groups, the plan terms regarding eligibility affected the magnitude of the eligible component in relation to total APBO.

TABLE 6.2 Components of APBO at Date of Adoption

	Percentage of APBO Attributable to:		
	Retirees	Actives Fully Eligible	Actives Not Yet Fully Eligible
Number of companies with:			
Less than 10%	1	5	1
10—19%	0	16	2
20—29%	1	5	7
30—39%	4	0	10
40—49%	8	0	3
50—59%	4	0	2
60—69%	5	0	0
Greater than 70%	3	0	1
	26	26	26
Average (mean) percentage by maturity:			
Highly mature companies	68%	11%	21%
Mature companies	45%	17%	38%
Immature companies	29%	20%	51%

The Vested Postretirement Benefit Obligation

The FASB proposal would require disclosure of the vested postretirement benefit obligation (VPBO) which is the actuarial present value of the obligation for retirees and their dependents plus the obligation for active employees computed using an assumption that all active employees immediately retire or terminate employment at the measurement date. Table 6.3 compares the VPBO to the APBO (both as of the end of the year that accrual accounting is adopted) for the hypothetical companies. Two comparisons are presented:

Total VPBO as a percentage of total APBO. In total, the VPBO is generally lower than the APBO because the VPBO does not contain the component of the obligation attributable to actives not yet eligible for any benefits. On the other hand, VPBO measures the benefits as though all participants that could immediately receive benefits would receive them starting immediately (including participants who could receive partial benefits but are not fully eligible), while the APBO measures only those benefits expected to be paid. VPBO as a percentage of total APBO is affected by both the number of actives eligible for any benefits and retirees in relation to the total plan population, and when payments are expected to begin (i.e., the retirement age assumption). Generally, the VPBO, as a percentage of the APBO, is greater for mature companies than for immature companies.

The eligible component of VPBO as a percentage of the eligible component of APBO. The retiree component is the same for both the APBO and VPBO. However, when looking at obligations for the group of active eligibles included in the APBO and VPBO, by definition, the VPBO is greater because it includes the estimated benefits that would be paid between the measurement date and the date at which benefit payments are expected to begin (i.e., expected retirement). In addition, the VPBO includes benefits that would be paid for actives eligible for partial benefits but not full benefits. Thus, the extent by which the eligible component of the VPBO is greater than the eligible component of the APBO is primarily affected by the retirement age assumption and the plan's eligibility provisions.

TABLE 6.3 Vested Postretirement Benefit Obligations (in Millions) — Hypothetical Companies

	Highly Mature Total Obligation	Highly Mature Eligible Component of Obligation	Immature Total Obligation	Immature Eligible Component of Obligation
APBO*	$103	$12	$25	$6
VPBO*	$ 84	$18	$15	$9
VPBO as a percentage of APBO	82%	150%	60%	150%

*At end of year of adoption.

Field Test Results

Table 6.4 summarizes results regarding the VPBO. The majority of Field Test companies approximated the results shown for the hypothetical companies. The VPBO as a percentage of the APBO averaged 83 percent, 68 percent, and 56 percent for the highly mature, mature, and immature Field Test companies, respectively. While the eligible component of the VPBO as a percentage of the eligible component of the APBO was 150 percent for both the highly mature and immature hypothetical companies, the actual Field Test companies exhibited wide diversity, ranging from 114 percent to over 200 percent.

TABLE 6.4 VPBO as a Percentage of APBO — End of Year of Adoption

Total Obligation:	Number of Companies
Less than 65%	7
65 — 74%	9
75 — 84%	4
Greater than 84%	6
	26
Eligible Component:*	
Less than 130%	2
130 — 149%	9
150 — 174%	8
175 — 199%	5
Greater than 199%	2
	26

* For some companies, VPBO includes obligations for actives eligible for partial benefits but not yet fully eligible.

The majority of the mature companies showed the VPBO as 65 to 74 percent of the APBO while most of the highly mature companies showed percentages greater than 75 percent. Almost all of the immature companies showed percentages of less than 65 percent. There were extreme cases where the VPBO for three companies exceeded 90 percent of the APBO and the VPBO for one company was less than 30 percent.

The eligible component of the VPBO as a percentage of the eligible component of the APBO did not exhibit any pattern by maturity, as defined for purposes of the Field Test. The relationship between the eligible component of the APBO and the eligible component of the VPBO depended more on the plans' eligibility criteria and when benefits are expected to begin (e.g., the retirement date assumption) than on demographics.

Obligations as a Multiple of Pay-As-You-Go

Because most companies currently record expense on a pay-as-you-go basis, it was concluded that a comparison between the APBO and benefit payments (pay-as-you-go) in the year of adoption may be helpful for comparative purposes. Table 6.5 presents this comparison for the hypothetical companies.

TABLE 6.5 APBO Compared to Annual Benefit Payments (Pay-As-You-Go) (in Millions) — Hypothetical Companies

	Highly Mature	Immature
APBO at date of adoption	$98.0	$22.6
Benefit payments in year of adoption	$ 6.2	$ 0.7
Multiple of APBO to benefit payments	15.8	32.3

Field Test Results

The APBO expressed as a multiple of benefit payments (pay-as-you-go) generally varied by maturity of the company as shown in table 6.6.

TABLE 6.6 APBO Compared to Benefit Payments (Pay-As-You-Go) in Year of Adoption

Companies with APBO as multiple of benefit payments:	Highly Mature	Mature	Immature	Total
Less than 16 times	3	2	0	5
17 to 32 times	6	7	1	14
Greater than 32 times	0	4	3	7
	9	13	4	26

Most highly mature Field Test companies showed a higher multiple of APBO to benefit payments than the highly mature hypothetical company, with only five companies with multiples under 16. In addition, seven companies had multiples in excess of 32, three of which were immature. The multiple of APBO to benefit payments is dependent on a number of factors including the demographic characteristics of active employees, the plan provisions, and the company's number of retirees. If, for example, there were no retirees currently and no current pay-as-you-go costs, the multiple would reach infinity.

Amortizing the Transition Obligation

Under the ED, the transition obligation would be equal to the present value of the benefits attributable to service prior to the date of adopting the statement (APBO) reduced by the fair value of plan assets, if any, and any accrued liability (asset) on the employer's balance sheet at that date. It was assumed that there were no plan assets or accrued liabilities (assets) for either hypothetical company at the date of adoption. Accordingly, the transition obligation determined at that date equals the APBO of $98 million and $22.6 million for the highly mature and immature hypothetical companies, respectively.

Under the ED, the transition obligation would generally be amortized on a straight-line basis over the average remaining service period (ARSP) to expected retirement for employees expected to receive benefits. If this period is less than 15 years, an employer may elect to use a 15-year period. If all or almost all plan participants are inactive, the average remaining life expectancy of the inactive participants would be used as the amortization period for the transition obligation with no 15-year option. (Refer to chapter 3 for a detailed discussion of the proposed requirements for recognizing and amortizing the transition obligation.)

Transition Amortization Periods

The ARSP to expected retirement for employees expected to receive benefits was compared with the ARSP under SFAS No. 87 (used for pension accounting). The two ARSPs differ because each is based on employees expected to receive benefits under the respective plan. Generally, pension benefits legally vest for employees who leave before retirement while health benefits do not. Accordingly, the ARSP for the hypothetical companies[2] under the ED (19.8 years) was approximately five years greater than the ARSP under SFAS No. 87. The ARSP under SFAS No. 87 was also compared to the ARSP to the date of full eligibility. For the hypothetical companies, the ARSP to eligibility was approximately the same as the ARSP under SFAS No. 87.

Field Test Results

The ARSP to expected retirement under the ED was greater than 15 years for almost all of the Field Test companies with the majority of Field Test companies having periods between 18 and 21 years. The opposite was true for the period to full eligibility with the majority of Field Test companies exhibiting periods to full eligibility of 15 years or less.

Table 6.7 shows these periods as well as the period under SFAS No. 87 reported by the Field Test companies. Table 6.8 provides a comparison of the various service periods analyzed. The results presented in these tables are based on combined periods for companies with more than one plan. One plan of one company had primarily inactive employees and the average remaining life expectancy of inactive participants was used for all periods. The 15-year optional period under the ED and SFAS No. 87 was not reflected in tables 6.7 and 6.8.

TABLE 6.7 ARSP for Field Test Companies as of Date of Adoption

Number of companies with:	ARSP to Expected Retirement	ARSP to Eligibility Date	ARSP Under SFAS No. 87
Less than 15 years	4	24	14
15—17.9 years	7	2	7
18—20.9 years	14	0	3
21 years and greater	1	0	0
	26	26	24*
Average (mean) number of years	17.8	12.9	14.5

* SFAS No. 87 periods were not supplied by all companies

TABLE 6.8 Comparison of ARSP in Year of Adoption

	ARSP to Expected Retirement vs. SFAS No. 87	ARSP to Eligibility Date vs. SFAS No. 87	ARSP to Expected Retirement vs. ARSP to Eligibility Date
Number of companies with an increase:			
Less than 2 years	4	7	1
2—3.9 years	7	1	7
4—5.9 years	9	0	10
6 years and greater	2	0	8
Number of companies with decrease:			
Less than 2 years	2	6	0
2—3.9 years	0	5	0
4—5.9 years	0	4	0
6 years and greater	0	1	0
	24*	24*	26

*SFAS No. 87 periods were not supplied by all companies.

In general, the ARSP to expected retirement was in excess of the optional 15-year transition amortization period proposed by the FASB. For the majority of the Field Test companies, the ARSP to expected retirement exceeded the ARSP to eligibility by more than four years (five years on average). The period to expected retirement was greater than the period under SFAS No. 87 (as reported by the Field Test companies) for almost all companies, with the period being longer by three years on average.

The Pay-As-You-Go Constraint

The FASB also proposes that the amortization of the transition obligation be no less rapid than recognition on a pay-as-you-go basis (the "pay-as-you-go constraint"). To ensure this, the proposed statement would require that amortization of the transition obligation be increased by the greater of "a" or "b" below:

a. the excess of the cumulative benefit payments for those retirees and actives fully eligible for benefits at date of adoption over the cumulative sum of amortization of the transition obligation and interest on the unpaid transition obligation; or

b. the excess of the cumulative benefit payments over the cumulative amount expensed (both from date of adoption of the statement).

The pay-as-you-go constraint would be operational only during the period during which the transition obligation is being amortized and would be adjusted to reflect any plan assets and accrued liabilities at transition.

Field Test Results

The pay-as-you-go constraint would be determined starting from the year of adoption of the statement. Increases in benefit payments resulting from plan amendments and actuarial losses (e.g., actual health care costs rising faster than assumed) would be reflected immediately in the benefit payments included in the test. For purposes of examining the impact of the pay-as-you-go constraint in the Field Test, it was assumed that there were no actuarial gains or losses or plan amendments. Thus, there was only one small plan within one Field Test company in which an additional transition amortization would have been required because of the pay-as-you-go constraint.

Observation: Under the ED, a company's actual expense for a particular year might have to be changed in the fourth quarter due to the application of the pay-as-you-go constraint. The constraint is to be determined based upon actual retiree health plan payments during the year. Although a company could estimate the impact of this constraint, final amounts may not be determinable until sometime after the measurement date for the company's financial statements. As a result, additional expense or income arising due to differences between estimated and actual payments in recognizing the effects of the pay-as-you-go constraint would need to be recognized as a fourth quarter adjustment.

Under the proposed test (a), employers may need to establish systems modifications to track cumulative payments during the transition period to participants *who were retired or fully eligible as of the date of adoption. Some observers of the FASB project have stated that the cost of maintaining this data may exceed the benefit of this test.*

Impact on Expense

Most companies currently expense retiree health costs as they are paid (pay-as-you-go).[3] Table 6.9 presents a comparison of expense under the ED for the year of adoption of accrual accounting to expense determined under pay-as-you-go accounting for the hypothetical companies.

TABLE 6.9 Expense in Year of Adoption (in Millions) — Hypothetical Companies

	Highly Mature	Immature
Expense under ED	$16.2	$4.4
Benefit payments (pay-as-you-go)	$6.2	$0.7
Multiple of first year expense to benefit payments	2.6	6.3

Field Test Results

Table 6.10 summarizes results regarding the multiple of first year expense under the ED to benefit payments (pay-as-you-go). As with many other variables examined in the Field Test, expense under the ED as a multiple of benefit payments varied with the ratio of active employees to retirees (excluding dependents). In the year of adoption, expense under the ED was between two and seven times the pay-as-you-go amounts for most Field Test companies (which predominantly are mature companies). However, some highly mature companies had multiples of accrued expense to benefit payments of under two times. Generally, immature companies had higher multiples of expense under the ED to benefit payments than mature companies. If there were no retirees currently and no current pay-as-you-go costs, the multiple would reach infinity.

While company demographics is a key indicator of the multiple of expense to benefit payments, other factors influence this multiple. Such factors include plan provisions capping the companies' promise (e.g., low lifetime maximums) and the assumed health care cost trend and discount rates.

TABLE 6.10 Expense under ED as Multiple of Benefit Payments (Pay-As-You-Go) in Year of Adoption

	Highly Mature	Mature	Immature	Total
Number of companies with:				
Less than 2.0 times	2	0	0	2
2.0—2.9 times	2	3	0	5
3.0—3.9 times	2	0	0	2
4.0—4.9 times	2	5	0	7
5.0—5.9 times	1	1	1	3
6.0—6.9 times	0	2	1	3
7 times and greater	0	2	2	4
	9	13	4	26

Expense Components

To understand the factors contributing to expense under the ED, it is important to focus on the components of expense. These components in the year of adoption for an unfunded plan include service cost, interest cost, and amortization of the transition obligation. Interest cost (primarily interest on the APBO) is usually the largest component of expense under accrual accounting. Retiree health benefits are discounted to their present values as of the measurement date and the present value needs to be "brought forward" each year by accruing one year's interest to account for the lapsing of a year. Unlike pensions, companies have generally not funded these obligations and, thus, there is no offset to this large interest cost component (by interest or earnings on plan assets). The components of expense in the year of adoption for the hypothetical companies, under the proposed statement, are shown in table 6.11.

TABLE 6.11 Components of Expense in Year of Adoption (in Millions) — Hypothetical Companies

	Highly Mature		Immature	
	Amount	Percent	Amount	Percent
Service cost	$ 2.4	15%	$1.2	27%
Interest cost	8.8	54	2.1	48
Amortization of the transition obligation	5.0	31	1.1	25
Total expense	$16.2	100%	$4.4	100%

Field Test Results

Table 6.12 summarizes results regarding components of expense for the Field Test companies. For mature and highly mature companies, the transition obligation would be even more significant than it is for the immature company. Thus, interest cost plus amortization of the transition obligation would comprise a larger portion of expense under the ED. The hypothetical highly mature company with 85 percent of accrued expense relating to the transition obligation (54 percent relating to interest cost and 31 percent relating to amortization) and 15 percent relating to service cost is generally representative of the highly mature companies in the Field Test. However, five companies showed interest cost plus transition amortization of over 90 percent of accrued expense.

The hypothetical immature company with 73 percent of expense under the ED relating to the transition obligation (48 percent relating to interest cost and 25 percent relating to amortization) and 27 percent relating to service cost is generally representative of the less mature companies included in the Field Test. For the immature company with a smaller APBO at transition, service cost is a more significant portion of total expense than it is for mature companies, often 25 percent or higher. However, interest cost is still relatively high, averaging 39 percent of total expense for the immature companies in the Field Test.

TABLE 6.12 Components of Expense as a Percentage of Total Expense in Year of Adoption*

	Highly Mature	Mature	Immature
Service Cost:			
Range	4 — 16%	11 — 25%	25 — 52%
Average	11%	18%	36%
Interest Cost:			
Range	49 — 65%	45 — 56%	34 — 46%
Average	54%	50%	39%
Transition Amortization:			
Range	30 — 45%	26 — 37%	14 — 33%
Average	35%	32%	25%

* Since only one plan of one company was affected by the pay-as-you-go constraint, the constraint was not considered in this presentation.

Interest cost was the most significant component of expense (exceeding 45 percent for all but three companies). Interest cost plus transition amortization exceeded 74 percent for all but three companies. The portion of expense attributable to amortization of the transition obligation will vary by the period used to amortize the obligation and thus is influenced by such factors as the demographic characteristics of the active employees and the expected retirement dates.

Pattern of Expense

Expense under the ED was projected for each Field Test company for 10 years following the date of adoption. The pattern of expense under the pay-as-you-go method was compared to the pattern under the ED. Table 6.13 shows the patterns of expense for the hypothetical companies.

TABLE 6.13 Patterns of Expense — Hypothetical Companies

	Multiple of Year 1			
	Highly Mature		Immature	
Year	Expense Under ED	Pay-As-You-Go	Expense Under ED	Pay-As-You-Go
1	1.0	1.0	1.0	1.0
5	1.3	1.2	1.5	1.6
10	1.8	1.5	2.5	2.9

Field Test Results

The pattern of expense during the first 10 years varied between mature and immature companies with expense under the ED generally increasing at a faster rate for the immature company than the mature company because a greater proportion of expense for the immature company is due to service and interest cost accruals. Similarly, the pay-as-you-go expense payments for the immature company generally increased more rapidly than for the mature company because of the projected increase in the number of retirees during the 10-year period. Table 6.14 summarizes the pattern of expense for the Field Test companies.

TABLE 6.14 Expense Under the ED and Pay-As-You-Go Expense in Years 5 and 10 as Multiple of First Year Amounts

	Expense Under ED		Pay-As-You-Go Expense	
	Year 5	Year 10	Year 5	Year 10
Number of companies with multiples of Year 1 amounts:				
1.0 — 1.4 times	25	7	11	4
1.5 — 1.9 times	1	16	11	5
2.0 — 2.4 times	0	3	4	5
2.5 — 2.9 times	0	0	0	6
3.0 times and greater	0	0	0	6
	26	26	26	26

About one fourth of the Field Test companies (mostly highly mature) showed a pattern of expense under the ED similar to the pattern of pay-as-you-go expense. For all but a few of the companies, pay-as-you-go expense increased at a faster rate than expense under the ED. As with other elements analyzed, the pattern of expense will vary depending on a number of factors including the company's demographic characteristics, plan provisions (e.g., lifetime maximums), and actuarial assumptions. Readers should also bear in mind that many factors such as plan amendments and changes in assumptions can affect future pay-as-you-go expense and expense under the ED. For purposes of the Field Test, gains and losses and plan amendments were not reflected in the computations of future benefit payments and expense.

Sensitivity to Assumptions

Obligations and expense under the proposed statement can vary significantly depending on the actuarial assumptions used to estimate future retiree health benefits. Under the ED, each significant assumption used to measure obligations and determine expense should reflect the best estimate with respect to that individual assumption. In addition, the ED would require that economic assumptions be consistent to the extent that they incorporate expectations of the same future economic conditions.

Health Care Cost Trend

Due to the substantial uncertainty about future health care costs, actual trends in health care benefits may vary from those assumed (see chapter 5). Since variations in the assumed health care cost trend rate can significantly affect results, expense for each Field Test company in the year of adoption was determined under a "best estimate" assumption as shown previously, as well as under two other assumed health care cost trend rates — labeled "optimistic" and "pessimistic" — selected by each company. The range of results shown in table 6.14 for the hypothetical companies using the optimistic and pessimistic assumptions was considered as one measure of sensitivity. The FASB, however, would require a different sensitivity disclosure. The proposed statement's disclosure requirements include reporting the impact of a one percentage point increase or decrease in the assumed health care cost trend rate on obligations and expense.

Table 6.15 presents a comparison of obligations at the date of adoption and expense in the year of adoption under alternate assumed health care cost trend rates for the hypothetical companies, with all other assumptions being the same as those used in the hypothetical illustrations earlier in this chapter. To illustrate the sensitivity based on the optimistic and pessimistic assumptions, the trend rates used are based on the economic research presented in chapter 5. To illustrate the sensitivity disclosure proposed in the ED, each future year's best estimate health care cost trend assumption was decreased by one percentage point (and, consequently for the hypothetical companies, the weighted-average rate). Since the optimistic and pessimistic rates were within one-half of one percentage point of the best estimate (on a weighted-average basis), the proposed disclosure with respect to the impact of a one percentage point change in the health care cost trend assumption resulted in obligations and expense amounts for the hypothetical companies outside of the range of results determined using the optimistic and pessimistic assumptions.

Observation: The weighted-average assumed health care cost trend rate would be disclosed in the financial statements under the ED. However, the proposed statement does not define the methodology to be used in determining the weighted average of these rates. For purposes of the Field Test, the weighted-average trend rate represents the constant annual increase that would be applied to expected benefit payments to produce the same total plan payments as that produced using cost trend rates which vary by year. The weighted-average trend rates that would be disclosed under the ED will vary by the methodology used to weigh rates. Even under the same methodology, other factors could influ-

ence the weighted trend rates disclosed such as particular plan provisions and company demographics.

TABLE 6.15 Obligations and Expense Under Alternate Health Care Cost Trend Assumptions (in Millions) — Hypothetical Companies

	\multicolumn{4}{c}{Highly Mature Health Care Cost Trend Assumption}
	FASB Sensitivity*	Optimistic	Best Estimate	Pessimistic
Weighted trend**	6.9%	7.3%	7.9%	8.5%
Obligations as of date of adoption:				
EPBO	$106	$112	$122	$134
APBO	$ 88	$ 92	$ 98	$106
Expense under ED in year of adoption	$ 14.3	$ 14.9	$ 16.2	$ 17.7
Multiple of expense under ED to benefit payments (pay-as-you-go)	2.3	2.4	2.6	2.9
Percentage change from best estimate:				
APBO	(10.2%)	(6.1%)	—	8.2%
Expense	(11.7%)	(8.0%)	—	9.3%
	\multicolumn{4}{c}{Immature Health Care Cost Trend Assumption}
	FASB Sensitivity*	Optimistic	Best Estimate	Pessimistic
Weighted trend**	6.9%	7.3%	7.9%	8.5%
Obligations as of date of adoption:				
EPBO	$30	$31	$35	$39
APBO	$20	$21	$23	$25
Expense under ED in year of adoption	$ 3.7	$ 4.0	$ 4.4	$ 5.0
Multiple of expense under ED to benefit payments (pay-as-you-go)	5.3	5.7	6.3	7.1
Percentage change from best estimate:				
APBO	(13.0%)	(8.7%)	—	8.7%
Expense	(15.9%)	(9.1%)	—	13.6%

*One percentage point decrease in best estimate.
**Chapter 5 contains a complete description of the alternate health care cost trend assumptions.

Field Test Results

All Field Test companies selected assumed health care cost trend rates which varied by year with higher rates in the earlier years. The weighted-average health care trend rates selected by each company varied from those used by the hypothetical companies. The range of rates selected by Field Test companies are shown in table 6.16.

TABLE 6.16 Field Test Companies' Weighted-Average Health Care Trend Assumptions

	Range of Weighted-Average Health Care Trend Assumptions	Median
Optimistic	5.7% — 9.8%	7.3%
Best estimate	6.2% — 11.3%	7.9%
Pessimistic	6.5% — 13.3%	8.5%
FASB Sensitivity (one percentage point decrease in best estimate)	5.2% — 10.5%	6.9%

Observation: The trends shown above were weighted-average rates, and the range between these weighted-average rates were affected by the nature of the benefits provided. The year-by-year assumed health care cost trend rates selected by each Field Test company did not show such a wide disparity. It is interesting to note that a one percentage point decrease in each year's best estimate rate does not necessarily result in a one percentage point decrease in the weighted-average rate due to the impact of such items as lifetime maximums.

In accordance with the requirements in the ED, most Field Test companies generally selected—on a weighted-average basis—an optimistic assumption that was approximately six-tenths of one percentage point below its best estimate rate and a pessimistic assumption that was approximately six-tenths of one percentage point above its best estimate. Table 6.17 summarizes the sensitivity analysis of health care cost trend rates.

For the most part, immature Field Test companies exhibited greater sensitivity to the assumed health care cost trend than mature companies. For highly mature companies, expense in the year of adoption using the optimistic trend rate was generally 5 percent to 10 percent below the best estimate, while for immature companies, expense was reduced by 9 percent to 13 percent. Similar patterns emerged using the pessimistic assumptions although the percentage increase in expense was somewhat higher. Thus it was concluded that because immature companies have relatively more active employees, with a longer period to apply the trend rate assumption, the immature company will be somewhat more sensitive to changes in the cost trend assumption than mature companies. In addition to the maturity of the company, the impact on expense under the ED of the alternate trend rates varied due to particular company plan provisions such as the level of lifetime maximums and the alternate trend rate selected.

TABLE 6.17   Impact of Alternate Health Care Cost Trend Rates on Obligations and Expense—Year of Adoption

Number of companies with an increase/decrease:	Optimistic APBO	Optimistic Expense (Decrease)	Pessimistic APBO	Pessimistic Expense (Increase)	FASB Sensitivity APBO	FASB Sensitivity Expense (Decrease)
Less than 5%	4	2	2	2	1	1
5.0 — 9.9%	17	16	13	11	8	6
10.0 — 14.9%	4	7	8	9	15	13
15.0 — 19.9%	1	1	1	2	2	5
Greater than 19.9%	0	0	2	2	0	1
	26	26	26	26	26	26

Alternate Health Care Cost Trend Approaches

Some observers of the FASB project have raised concerns that the results of the measurements that would be required under the ED would not be reliable due to the fact that they would involve the projection of health care costs for many years into the future. Various alternative approaches have been suggested to try to mitigate the issue of reliability, including the following:

Nonprojected approach.   Current per capita cost levels could be viewed as a minimum estimate of future costs (i.e., a 0 percent cost trend assumption). Some observers of the FASB project believe that under this approach, measurements of obligations and expense under accrual accounting would not have to rely on projections of future trends that they view as unreliable and speculative. Because health care costs are expected to rise and large actuarial losses may arise using this approach, some observers might deem it appropriate to immediately recognize such losses.

Some would reject the nonprojected approach, questioning whether discounting the obligation could be deemed to be appropriate under a method that did not project future increases in health care costs. In other words, it might not be internally consistent to remove inflation from the cost trend but anticipate inflation in setting the discount rate, thus discounting current costs.

Nonprojected/nondiscounted approach. The FASB considered an approach that would be based on current per capita costs but no discounting (i.e., a 0 percent cost trend assumption with a 0 percent discount rate). Such an approach would be based on a premise that all future projections of inflation are unreliable and there should be a linkage between the health care cost trend rate and the discount rate. However, some would conclude that this approach is an implicit rather than explicit approach to selecting assumptions. The Board concluded that each assumption should be based on a "best estimate" of future events.

General inflation approach. Since health costs have historically exceeded the rate of general inflation, some believe that the minimum estimate of future costs could be based on an assumption of future general inflation (an assumed 4½ percent cost trend rate, for example). Proponents of this approach believe that it would mitigate some concerns regarding reliability, while still adding a measure of future cost increases. Again, this would be considered by some as an implicit approach.

Medical inflation approach. Since health cost increases due to changing technology and utilization patterns may be viewed as the most unreliable component of the assumed health care cost trend rate, some observers of the FASB project would base the assumed cost trend rate on expected medical price inflation (a 6 percent trend rate, for example), rather than an all-encompassing weighted-average health care cost trend rate (e.g., 7.9 percent). Proponents of this approach would emphasize that changes due to non-price factors are difficult to project based on past experience. Some would conclude, however, that a best estimate of these factors is more appropriate under an explicit approach.

The above alternative cost trend approaches were modeled for the hypothetical companies and for certain Field Test companies. As expected, these projections resulted in dramatic decreases in expense under accrual accounting in the year of adoption. Estimating the impact of these alternate approaches in later years depends on the projection of actual future increases in health care costs and on the approach used to account for actuarial gains and losses.

The estimated impact of the alternative health care cost trend approaches in the year of adoption on the hypothetical companies is shown in table 6.18.

TABLE 6.18 Alternate Health Care Trend Approaches — Hypothetical Companies

	ED Approach ($millions)	Percentage Change from ED Approach			
		Nonpro-jected Approach	Nonpro-jected/ Nondis-counted Approach	General Inflation Approach	Medical Inflation Approach
Assumed trend rate	7.9%	0%	0%	4.5%	6%
Assumed discount rate	9.25%	9.25%	0%	9.25%	9.25%
Highly mature:					
APBO at date of adoption	$98	(53.1%)	15.3%	(31.8%)	(21.0%)
Expense in year of adoption	$16.2	(58.0%)	(45.0%)	(35.5%)	(23.2%)
Immature:					
APBO at date of adoption	$23	(64.9%)	21.8%	(41.0%)	(27.3%)
Expense in year of adoption	$ 4.4	(68.9%)	(31.5%)	(43.0%)	(27.6%)

Observation: Under a nonprojected/nondiscounted approach, the APBO at the date of adoption could be somewhat higher or lower than under the best estimate approach in the ED, depending on the spread between the assumed health care cost trend and discount rates. However, expense in the year of adoption will be significantly less under this approach than under the ED because there is no interest cost using a nondiscounted approach. Generally, any increased service cost and transition amortization components of first year expense under a nonprojected/nondiscounted approach will be less than the eliminated interest cost component.

Discount Rate

The assumed discount rate tends to counterbalance the effect of the health care cost trend assumption. The higher the discount rate, the lower the present value of projected obligations. The opposite is true for the assumed health care cost trend rate. Table 6.19 shows the impact of a one percentage point increase in the discount rate assumption on the hypothetical companies' obligations and expense.

Field Test Results

The discount rates selected by the participating Field Test companies, using the guidance in the ED, ranged from 7.5 percent to 11 percent. However, the impact of a one percentage point change in the discount rate depends not only on the rate selected, but also on the relative maturity of the population. As with respect to the assumed health care cost trend rate, changing the discount rate will have a greater impact on the immature company. A one percentage point increase in the discount rate decreased the APBO and expense for the Field Test companies in the year of adoption as shown in table 6.20.

TABLE 6.19 Impact of One Percentage Point Increase in Discount Rate on Obligations and Expense — Hypothetical Companies (in Millions)

	\multicolumn{4}{c}{Highly Mature}
	Discount Rate Based on ED (9.25%)	Discount Rate Based on ED + 1% (10.25%)	Decrease	Percentage Change
Obligations as of date of adoption:				
EPBO	$122	$106	$16	(13.1%)
APBO	$ 98	$ 88	$10	(10.2%)
Expense in year of adoption	$ 16.2	$ 15.1	$ 1.1	(6.8%)
Multiple of expense to benefit payments (pay-as-you-go)	2.6	2.4	—	(7.7%)

	\multicolumn{4}{c}{Immature}
	Discount Rate Based on ED (9.25%)	Discount Rate Based on ED + 1% (10.25%)	Decrease	Percentage Change
Obligations as of date of adoption:				
EPBO	$35	$30	$5	(14.3%)
APBO	$23	$20	$3	(13.0%)
Expense in year of adoption	$ 4.4	$ 3.9	$0.5	(11.4%)
Multiple of expense to benefit payments (pay-as-you-go)	6.3	5.6	—	(11.1%)

TABLE 6.20 Impact of One Percentage Point Increase in Discount Rate on Obligations and Expense—Year of Adoption

Number of companies with decreases:	APBO Highly Mature	APBO Mature	APBO Immature	Expense Highly Mature	Expense Mature	Expense Immature
Less than 7%	1	0	0	4	3	0
7.0 — 9.9%	2	2	0	4	6	1
10.0 — 12.9%	4	7	1	1	4	2
13% and greater	2	4	3	0	0	1
	9	13	4	9	13	4

Percent decrease by maturity of Field Test companies	APBO Range	APBO Average	Expense Range	Expense Average
Highly Mature	6.6 to 14.2	11.0	1.3 to 10.3	7.0
Mature	9.3 to 14.7	12.0	5.6 to 11.4	8.4
Immature	12.5 to 19.1	14.9	8.9 to 17.5	12.5

Obligations and expense for immature companies generally decreased by a greater extent due to a one percentage point increase in the discount rate than for mature Field Test companies. A one percentage point increase in the discount rate resulted in a greater reduction to the APBO than to first year expense because the higher interest rate is applied to a lower APBO in computing interest cost. However, the impact varied by factors other than maturity, including the discount rate selected.

The majority of Field Test companies selected discount rate assumptions that were between one to two percentage points higher than the weighted-average health care cost trend rate based on the best estimate assumptions in the year of adoption. In the early years after adoption, the assumed health care cost trend rates were higher than the assumed discount rates, while in later years the opposite was true.

Alternative Discount Rate Assumption

Because retiree health obligations are generally unfunded, some observers of the FASB project believe that the discount rate assumption should not be based on a hypothetical settlement of the obligation as called for under the ED. Generally, there are no settlement vehicles currently available for retiree health obligations that are similar to the annuities used to settle pension benefits. As a result, there are those who believe that since company funds will be used to settle the obligation, the discount rate should be based on a company's specific cost of borrowing or cost of capital. Accordingly, to measure the impact of using a company-specific discount assumption, each Field Test company generally selected a "company-specific" discount rate.

The FASB, however, believes that the funding of benefits should not affect the selection of the discount rate. The Board also concluded that an obligation to provide specified postretirement benefits should not be valued differently by different employers simply because their internal rates of return or assumed returns on plan assets differ. Some would also state that using a company-specific rate is improper because a company with poor credit (a high borrowing rate) could have a lower retiree health obligation than a company with a low borrowing rate.

Table 6.21 illustrates the impact on the determination of the hypothetical companies' obligations and expense in the year of adoption of using an assumed company-specific discount rate of 12.0 percent rather than the discount rate of 9.25 percent based on the guidance in the ED.

Observation: Some observers of the FASB project believe that the discount rate should not be changed annually—as it is for pensions under SFAS No. 87—based on yearly fluctuations in interest rates. They argue that short-term swings in a long-term rate produce unnecessary volatility and therefore should not be considered unless the change in interest rates is indicative of the long-term trend. For unfunded retiree health plans, the impact of changing the discount rate would not be offset by changes in the value of plan assets. The FASB, however, concluded that the selection of the discount rate for retiree health and other postretirement benefits should not be conceptually different than for pension plans. For purposes of this analysis, the trend rate was not changed.

Field Test Results

Company-specific discount rates selected by Field Test companies ranged from 9 percent to 15 percent, with most companies' company-specific rate about one percentage point to three percentage points above the discount rate selected based on the guidance in the ED. Three companies used rates below 10 percent and three companies used rates in excess of 12 percent.

TABLE 6.21 Impact of Alternate Discount Rate Assumption on Obligations and Expense — Hypothetical Companies (in Millions)

	Highly Mature			
	Discount Rate Under ED (9.25%)	Company-Specific Discount Rate (12%)	Decrease	Percentage Change
Obligations as of date of adoption:				
EPBO	$122	$83	$39	(32.0%)
APBO	$ 98	$74	$24	(24.5%)
Expense under ED in year of adoption	$ 16.2	$13.6	$2.6	(16.0%)
Multiple of expense to benefit payments (pay-as-you-go)	2.6	2.2	—	(15.4%)

	Immature			
	Discount Rate Under ED (9.25%)	Company-Specific Discount Rate (12%)	Decrease	Percentage Change
Obligations as of date of adoption:				
EPBO	$35	$21	$14	(40.0%)
APBO	$23	$15	$ 8	(34.8%)
Expense under ED in year of adoption	$ 4.4	$ 3.2	$ 1.2	(27.3%)
Multiple of expense to benefit payments (pay-as-you-go)	6.3	4.6	—	(27.0%)

The impact of using a company-specific rate depended heavily on the variation from the rate used under the ED and was less dependent on the relative maturity of the companies (though, as noted earlier, the impact of changing assumptions has relatively greater effect on results for the immature company). For example, one company increased its discount rate by six-tenths of one percentage point, decreasing its APBO at adoption by 8.3 percent and its first year expense by 6.1 percent. Another company increased its discount rate by five percentage points, decreasing its APBO at adoption by about 40 percent and its first year expense by about 30 percent. The impact on obligations and expense under the ED of using a company-specific rate is shown in table 6.22.

TABLE 6.22 Impact of Company-Specific Discount Rate on Obligations and Expense in Year of Adoption

	Increase in Discount Rate from ED Rate		
Decrease in:	Less than Two Percentage Points	Two to Three Percentage Points	Greater than Three Percentage Points
APBO at date of adoption	4.8 to 17.7%	25.1 to 34.3%	27.9 to 41.6%
Expense in year of adoption	2.8 to 14.5%	20.4 to 31.7%	16.9 to 29.6%

Overall, the use of a company-specific discount rate decreased the APBO at date of adoption by 5 percent to 42 percent and expense in the year of adoption by 3 percent to 32 percent. As shown, the impact of using a company-specific rate depended heavily on the variation from the rate used under the ED. Generally, the greater the change in the discount rate the greater the impact on obligations and expense.

Analysis of Alternate Accounting Approaches

To analyze the impact of alternative approaches to various provisions contained in the ED, two key elements contributing to expense were isolated and examined—the attribution period and amortization of the transition obligation.

In order to examine the impact of each of the elements separately, the pay-as-you-go constraint requirements of the proposed statement (discussed earlier in this chapter) were not recognized for purposes of this analysis.

Impact of Attribution Period

The ED requires that companies use a single attribution method based on the terms of the plan to determine retiree health expense. Under this method (which the FASB calls a benefit/years-of-service approach), the cost of a participant's benefits are allocated to individual years of service. Where benefits are not defined by a plan formula, costs would be allocated to service under the ED from date-of-hire to the date the employee is fully eligible for benefits (the attribution period). Many observers have argued for the alternative that costs should be spread from an employee's date of hire to the expected date of retirement (the full-service period).

The attribution period is used to attribute (or assign) costs to individual years of service and affects the allocation of the present value of the EPBO between the past and future service and, thus, can impact the APBO and service cost.

Using a full-service period approach changes the transition obligation. Under the ED, the transition obligation includes 100 percent of the obligation for retirees and eligibles plus a proportionate amount for actives not yet eligible. Under a full-service period approach, the transition obligation would be based on the obligation for retirees plus a proportionate amount for all active employees, creating a lower transition obligation and lower interest cost. A full-service period approach would generally spread costs (i.e., service cost) over a longer period.

Observation: At one point in the FASB's deliberations, a majority of Board members supported a full-service attribution period. As expressed in the "Alternate Views" section of the ED, two Board members continue to believe that a full-service period approach should be used for plans that do not have a benefit formula that directly defines benefits earned in exchange for service in specific years. In this view, the agreement that the employee will receive benefits after retirement in exchange for service prior to retirement is best reflected by attributing the cost of retiree benefits over all years of employee service to the expected retirement date.

Table 6.23 presents the impact on obligations and expense for the hypothetical companies using a full-service period approach.

Field Test Results

The impact of using a full-service period approach would generally be greater for an immature company than for a highly mature company, as shown by the hypothetical illustrations. In addition, the impact of using a full-service period approach depends on other factors such as the plan's eligibility provisions and the early retirement assumption.

For more than one-half of the Field Test companies, the full-service period approach reduced first year obligations and expense, and expense cumulatively for the first 10 years by 4 to 10 percent.

TABLE 6.23 Full-Service Attribution Period (in Millions) — Hypothetical Companies

	Highly Mature			Immature		
	ED Approach*	Full-Service Period	Percentage Difference	ED Approach*	Full-Service Period	Percentage Difference
Obligations at date of adoption:						
EPBO	$122	$122	0%	$35	$35	0%
APBO	$ 98	$ 93	(5%)	$23	$20	(13%)
Expense:						
Year of adoption	$ 16.2	$ 15.2	(6%)	$ 4.4	$ 3.9	(11%)
Cumulative - 10 years	$217.4	$199.0	(8%)	$73.3	$64.0	(13%)
Multiple of expense to benefit payments:						
Year of adoption	2.6	2.5	(4%)	6.3	5.6	(11%)
Cumulative - 10 years	2.8	2.6	(7%)	6.0	5.2	(13%)

*Costs attributed to service from employee's date of hire to full eligibility date.

The impact on obligations and expense for the Field Test companies of using a full-service approach in the year of adoption and the cumulative impact on expense over 10 years is shown in table 6.24.

Impact of Amortization of the Transition Obligation
Amortization Period
Altering the period over which the transition obligation is amortized can have a significant impact on the level of expense under the ED. However, the transition amortization is only one component of expense. Thus, for example, changing the amortization period from 15 years to 30 years does not decrease expense by one-half; it only decreases the portion of expense attributable to the transition amortization by one-half. In addition many Field Test companies have average remaining service periods of about 20 years, so permitting a 30-year period would decrease annual transition amortization by one-third.

TABLE 6.24 Comparison of Obligations and Expense Under Full-Service Attribution Period and ED Attribution Period

	Highly Mature	Mature	Immature	Total
APBO at Date of Adoption				
Number of companies with decrease:				
Less than 4%	3	1	0	4
4 — 6.9%	5	0	0	5
7 — 9.9%	1	7	3	11
10 — 12.9%	0	3	0	3
13 — 15.9%	0	1	0	1
16% and greater	0	1	1	2
	9	13	4	26
Average decrease in APBO	4.4%	10.1%	12.8%	8.5%
Expense in Year of Adoption				
Number of companies with decrease:				
Less than 4%	5	2	0	7
4 — 6.9%	3	4	1	8
7 — 9.9%	1	3	1	5
10 — 12.9%	0	3	1	4
13 — 15.9%	0	0	0	0
16% and greater	0	1	1	2
	9	13	4	26
Average decrease in expense	4.0%	8.3%	11.1%	7.3%
Expense — 10-Year Cumulative				
Number of companies with decrease:				
Less than 4%	5	1	0	6
4 — 6.9%	3	5	1	9
7 — 9.9%	1	3	1	5
10 — 12.9%	0	2	1	3
13 — 15.9%	0	1	0	1
16% and greater	0	1	1	2
	9	13	4	26
Average decrease in cumulative expense	4.3%	8.3%	10.7%	7.3%

Observation: Some observers of the FASB project take the view that immediate recognition of the entire transition obligation should be permitted—either through a cumulative catch-up charge against net income or by directly charging stockholders' equity. The potential impact of such approaches is presented in chapter 8.

Table 6.25 illustrates the impact on the hypothetical companies of amortizing the transition obligation ($98 million for the highly mature company and $23 million for the immature company) on a straight-line basis over the alternate amortization periods included in the Field Test.

TABLE 6.25 Amortizing the Transition Obligation on a Straight-Line Basis — Impact on Expense (in Millions) — Hypothetical Companies

	Highly Mature		Immature	
	Year of Adoption	Cumulative —10 Years	Year of Adoption	Cumulative —10 Years
Amortization Period ARSP to:	Expense / Percent Change*	Expense / Percent Change*	Expense / Percent Change*	Expense / Percent Change*
Expected retirement**	$16.2 —	$217 —	$4.4 —	$73.3 —
Eligibility date***	18.1 11.7%	236 8.8%	4.9 11.4%	77.7 6.0%
15 years	17.8 9.9%	233 7.4%	4.8 9.1%	76.9 4.9%
30 years	14.5 (10.5%)	201 (7.4%)	4.1 (6.8%)	69.4 (5.3%)

*Represents percent change from ARSP to expected retirement.

**For hypothetical companies, ARSP to expected retirement (19.8 years) would be used under ED since it is longer than 15 years.

***ARSP to eligibility date is 14.8 years for hypothetical companies.

Field Test Results

The following amortization periods were analyzed for the Field Test companies:

ARSP to expected retirement. If the transition obligation were to be amortized over the ARSP to expected retirement date (without recognition of the 15-year optional period), expense would have increased for only five companies since, for all other companies, the 15-year optional period was less than the period to expected retirement for all plans. For three of these five companies, the period to expected retirement was less than 15 years for all of their plans. Since the period to expected retirement was close to 15 years for all but one of these companies, the impact on expense of the 15-year option was less than 3 percent for most of these companies.

ARSP to eligibility date. The difference between the ARSP to expected retirement and eligibility date is primarily driven by the company's assumptions as to the retirement date and the eligibility criteria under the plan. If the transition obligation were to be amortized over the ARSP to eligibility date (without recognition of the 15-year optional period) rather than expected retirement, the first year expense would increase by 4 percent to 31 percent for the Field Test companies. Four companies experienced increases of less than 7 percent in first year expense, four had increases of more than 24 percent. The ARSP to eligibility date was less than 15 years for all but a few Field Test companies. If a 15-year optional period had been recognized for the ARSP to eligibility date, the increase in expense would have been less.

30-year optional amortization period. If the FASB were to allow a 30-year amortization period (as opposed to the 15-year optional period proposed in the ED), most of the Field Test companies would have experienced a reduction in the annual amortization of the transition obligation from about 30 percent to 50 percent (with companies using a 15-year period under the ED for all plans exhibiting the 50 percent reduction in amortization). The effect of this reduced amortization on annual expense depends on both the magnitude of the transition obligation and the period used to amortize the obligation under the ED with the period being the primary determinant. As shown in table 6.26, in the year of adoption, the 30-year amortization period reduced first year expense under the ED for the Field Test companies by 2 percent to 20 percent.

Overall, the impact on expense of increasing the period of amortization depended more heavily on the ARSP used to amortize expense under the ED than the maturity of the companies. However, expense under the ED in the year of adoption for two immature companies with relatively low transition obligations and long ARSPs, decreased by less than 8 percent. Several mature and highly mature companies and one immature company with average remaining service periods of less than 16 years had first year expense reductions of greater than 16 percent using a 30-year period.

Observation: The use of a longer amortization period for some companies may not be as significant as illustrated for the Field Test companies because of the proposed pay-as-you-go constraint discussed earlier in this chapter.

TABLE 6.26 Amortization of Transition Obligation Over 30 Years Compared to Amortization Under ED*

	No.	ARSP Under ED	Average Decrease in Amortization	Average Decrease in Expense Year of Adoption	Cumulative— 10 Years
Number of companies with decrease in amortization:					
Less than 35%	7	greater than 19.2 years	30.1%	8.3%	6.4%
35 — 45%	10	16.0 to 19.2	39.9%	12.6%	9.7%
Greater than 45%	8	less than 16 years	48.8%	17.6%	14.5%
	25**				

*Amortization under ED recognizes 15-year optional amortization period.
**Excludes one company affected by pay-as-you-go constraint.

Mortgage-Type Amortization Technique

The ED would require that the transition obligation be amortized to expense on a straight-line basis. However, for pension funding purposes, prior service costs have traditionally been amortized on an actuarial basis using an approach that produces a level amount of principal plus interest, similar to a conventional mortgage. Similarly, the impact of using a mortgage-type approach to amortize the transition obligation was modeled, using a reverse-sum-of-the-digits method. Under this method, the transition obligation was amortized according to the following 20-year schedule:

$$\text{Year } 1 = 1/210$$
$$\text{Year } 2 = 2/210$$
$$\bullet$$
$$\bullet$$
$$\bullet$$
$$\text{Year } 20 = 20/210$$

Observation: The FASB rejected the use of mortgage-type amortization techniques for pension prior service costs and transition amounts under SFAS No. 87. For postretirement benefits, the Board found no justification for a different approach than used in SFAS No. 87. In addition, the FASB notes in the ED that funding should not drive the accounting and that transition obligations for postretirement benefits are inherently different from pension prior service costs (i.e., the transition obligation for postretirement benefits is largely unrecognized service and interest cost, not the unamortized costs of plan amendments).

Expense under the mortgage-type transition approach method would produce a lower level of amortization than the ED in the early years after adoption. However, just like a conventional mortgage, "principal" payments rise each year. As a result, expense in later years would be greater under this approach. Table 6.27 shows expense for the hypothetical companies determined using the above pattern of amortizing the transition obligation similar to a mortgage-type amortization approach.

TABLE 6.27 Mortgage-Type Transition Amortization Approach—Impact on Expense (in Millions) — Hypothetical Companies

	Highly Mature		Immature	
	Year of Adoption	Cumulative 10 Years	Year of Adoption	Cumulative 10 Years
Straight-line (ED)	$16.2	$217	$4.4	$73.3
Mortgage-type approach	$11.7	$194	$3.4	$67.8
Percent decrease	28%	11%	23%	8%

Field Test Results

As with other approaches that affect amortization of the transition obligation, the impact of using a mortgage-type amortization approach is greatest in the early years after transition for mature companies with large transition obligations. In addition, the impact of this approach is greater for companies with shorter amortization periods (e.g., 16 years versus 20 years). For example, several highly mature Field Test companies showed first year expense reductions of 35 percent and over using this approach while other highly mature companies had reductions under 30 percent. Overall, first year expense was reduced from 13 percent to 38 percent as shown in table 6.28. However, these expense reductions decrease annually under a mortgage approach so that the 10-year cumulative reduction in expense was about 3 percent to 22 percent.

TABLE 6.28 Expense under Mortgage-Type Amortization Approach Compared to Expense under the ED*

	Reduction in Expense	
	Year of Adoption	Cumulative—10 Years
Maturity of the company:		
Highly mature	28.1% to 37.9%	11.5% to 21.8%
Mature	24.3% to 33.9%	8.7% to 17.7%
Immature	13.2% to 30.4%	2.8% to 14.3%
ARSP to expected retirement:		
Under 19 Years	25.7% to 37.9%	10.2% to 21.8%
Over 19 Years	13.2% to 29.0%	2.8% to 15.3%

*Amortization under the ED reflects amortization over ARSP or 15 years if greater.

Alternate "Grandfathering" Transition Approach

In order to mitigate the impact of switching to accrual accounting, other approaches that delay recognition have been suggested. One alternative approach to transition could be to continue to expense under the pay-as-you-go method for retirees—or perhaps retirees and active employees fully eligible for benefits—at transition and apply the provisions of the ED to only active employees (or active employees not yet fully eligible) as of the transition date (and later). This could be viewed as an approach similar to that often used by Congress when new laws are passed—referred to as "grandfathering." While to some observers this approach may not be justifiable from a conceptual accounting viewpoint, other observers of the FASB project believe that practical considerations should be addressed in selecting a transition approach. However, since the "grandfathering" approach delays recognition of the retiree obligation—perhaps the most definite and reliable component of the APBO—others would reject this approach.

To illustrate one "grandfathering" approach that could be selected, the pay-as-you-go method was continued for retirees as of the transition date for the Field Test companies and the full-service period was used to attribute costs to years of service for active employees. Table 6.29 presents the impact of this approach on the hypothetical companies. The pay-as-you-go constraint requirements proposed by the FASB were not considered in developing this illustration.

118   *Retiree Health Benefits*

Observation: If a "grandfathering" approach were adopted, companies would need to consider whether systems modifications will be needed to track benefit payments to those who were retired (or fully eligible) at the date of transition.

TABLE 6.29 Alternative "Grandfathering" Transition Amortization Approach—Impact on Expense (in Millions) — Hypothetical Companies

	Highly Mature		Immature	
	Year of Adoption	Cumulative 10 Years	Year of Adoption	Cumulative 10 Years
Exposure draft	$16.2	$217	$4.4	$73.3
"Grandfathering" approach	$12.1	$176	$3.6	$61.7
Percent decrease	25%	19%	18%	16%

Field Test Results

Because this "grandfathering" method delays the recognition of interest cost on the transition obligation for retirees until payments are made, those with a large number of retirees would generally be more affected than those with few retirees. However, the impact on expense also depends on the relationship between amortization of the transition obligation and benefit payments to retirees. The impact on expense would be less where payments to retirees are greater than amortization of the obligation associated with retirees. Thus, as shown in table 6.30, some highly mature Field Test companies had first year expense reductions of over 30 percent and other highly mature Field Test companies had first year expense reductions of less than 22 percent. The effect on immature Field Test companies was generally lower, with all having first year expense reduced by 22 percent or less.

TABLE 6.30 Expense under Alternative "Grandfathering" Transition Amortization Approach Compared to Expense under the ED

	Reduction in Expense	
	Year of Adoption	Cumulative—10 Years
Highly mature	7.0% to 41.6%	4.2% to 31.4%
Mature	14.9% to 36.2%	4.3% to 24.7%
Immature	16.1% to 22.0%	13.5% to 18.9%

Observation: Generally, the grandfathering approach produced a decrease in first year expense for the Field Test companies. However, there may be certain circumstances under which this approach may increase expense. In addition, this approach may be difficult to apply to a funded situation.

Impact on Recorded Liabilities and Assets

Under the FASB proposal, a liability would be recorded if the cumulative expense charged to income exceeds the cumulative amounts funded or paid (accrued liability). In addition, five years after application of the proposed standard, an additional liability might need to be recorded so that the total liability recorded (including accrued liability) would not be less than the excess of the APBO for retirees and actives fully eligible for benefits over the total fair value of plan assets (see chapter 3).

Table 6.31 presents the amount of accrued liability that would be recorded by the hypothetical companies for the years following the application of the proposed standard. Also shown is the amount of additional liability that would be recorded based on the five-year delay in the minimum liability provisions under the ED (i.e., the minimum liability would be recorded starting in year 6).

No plan amendments increasing benefit levels or actuarial losses were assumed in developing table 6.31 and for purposes of the Field Test. In practice, if actuarial losses or plan amendments are significant, the impact of the minimum liability requirements could be of greater significance than that demonstrated below.

Field Test Results

For the hypothetical highly mature company, the accrued liability in year 6 was 73 percent of the APBO for retirees and active employees fully eligible, but by year 9 the minimum liability provisions in the ED were inoperative since the accrued liability was greater than the unfunded APBO for retirees and active employees fully eligible. This pattern generally held for highly mature Field Test companies, with some exceeding 10 years before the minimum liability becomes inoperative.

Because a large portion of plan participants of the immature company are active employees not yet eligible, accrued liabilities build relatively faster than for the mature company. As a result the accrued liability of the immature hypothetical company exceeded the unfunded APBO for retirees and active employees fully eligible by the end of year 5. This pattern generally held for the immature companies.

TABLE 6.31 Accrued and Minimum Liability Provisions (in Millions)—Hypothetical Companies

HIGHLY MATURE

Year	Accrued Expense[1]	Benefit Payments[2]	Accrued Liability[3]	Unfunded APBO for Retirees and Eligibles[4]	Liability Reflected on Balance Sheet[5]	Intangible Asset and Additional Liability[6]
1	$16.2	$6.2	$ 10.0	$ 80.4	$ 10.0	$ —
2	17.2	6.5	20.7	83.4	20.7	—
3	18.2	6.9	32.0	87.1	32.0	—
4	19.3	7.2	44.1	90.5	44.1	—
5	20.6	7.5	57.2	94.3	57.2	—
6	21.9	7.8	71.3	98.2	98.2	27.0
7	23.5	8.2	86.6	102.8	102.8	16.2
8	25.0	8.6	103.0	109.0	109.0	6.0
9	26.8	8.9	120.9	114.7	120.9	—
10	28.7	9.3	140.3	121.4	140.3	—

IMMATURE

Year	Accrued Expense[1]	Benefit Payments[2]	Accrued Liability[3]	Unfunded APBO for Retirees and Eligibles[4]	Liability Reflected on Balance Sheet[5]	Intangible Asset and Additional Liability[6]
1	$ 4.4	$0.7	$ 3.7	$ 13.1	$ 3.7	—
2	5.0	0.8	7.9	14.7	7.9	—
3	5.5	0.9	12.5	16.7	12.5	—
4	6.1	1.0	17.6	18.7	17.6	—
5	6.7	1.1	23.2	20.9	23.2	—
6	7.4	1.2	29.4	23.3	29.4	—
7	8.2	1.4	36.2	26.0	36.2	—
8	9.0	1.6	43.6	29.7	43.6	—
9	10.0	1.8	51.8	33.1	51.8	—
10	11.0	2.0	60.8	37.1	60.8	—

[1]Accrued Expense refers to the annual accrued expense under the proposed accounting requirements.
[2]Benefit Payments refers to actual cash outlay used to pay retiree benefits.
[3]Accrued Liability is the unfunded accrued expense, which is the cumulative difference between Accrued Expense and Benefit Payments.
[4]Unfunded APBO for Retirees and Eligibles is the actuarially determined present value of benefits expected to be paid after retirement for retirees and active employees fully eligible to receive benefits in excess of the fair value of plan assets. This unfunded amount represents the "minimum liability" as defined by the FASB.

[5]Liability Reflected on Balance Sheet is the amount that would be reported as a liability on the balance sheet equal to the Accrued Liability or, starting five years after the effective date of the proposed accrual accounting requirements, the greater of the Accrued Liability or the APBO for Retirees and Eligibles.
[6]The Additional Liability is, when the minimum liability requirements are effective, the excess of the APBO for Retirees and Eligibles over the Accrued Liability. Intangible Asset is the contra account to the Additional Liability.

The accrued liability as a percentage of the APBO for retirees and eligibles at the end of the fifth year following adoption (year 6) for the Field Test companies is shown in table 6.32.

TABLE 6.32 Accrued Liability on Balance Sheet as Percentage of APBO for Retirees and Eligibles at End of Sixth Year

Number of companies with percentage	Highly Mature	Mature	Immature	Total
Less than 60%	2	0	0	2
60 — 70%	4	1	0	5
70 — 80%	1	1	0	2
80 — 90%	2	5	0	7
90 — 100%	0	2	1	3
100 — 125%	0	3	1	4
Greater than 125%	0	1	2	3
	9	13	4	26

An additional liability would be required to be recorded five years after adoption of the ED (year 6) for 73 percent of the Field Test companies. Only four mature and three immature companies would not be required to record an additional liability.

An analysis of the year in which the accrued balance sheet liability exceeds the APBO for retirees and eligibles is shown in table 6.33.

TABLE 6.33 Analysis of Year Minimum Liability Provisions Become Inoperative under ED

Number of companies for which the accrued liability exceeds the APBO for retirees and eligibles:	Highly Mature	Mature	Immature	Total
Year 6 and prior	0	4	3	7
Years 7 — 8	2	5	1	8
Years 9 — 10	2	3	0	5
Later than 10 years	5	1	0	6
	9	13	4	26

An additional minimum liability would not be required to be recorded after 10 years following application of the ED for about one-half of the highly mature companies, and all of the immature companies. This analysis assumes no actuarial losses or plan amendments during this period. Actuarial losses or plan amendments increasing obligations would lengthen the number of years for the minimum liability provision to become inoperative, while the reverse is true for actuarial gains and plan amendments decreasing obligations.

Alternate Minimum Liability Basis

The impact of the minimum liability provisions contained in the ED was examined based on the unfunded APBO for retirees only and the unfunded accumulated obligation for all actives and retirees using a 0 percent health care cost trend assumption (with discounting). Some observers of the FASB project believe that using the APBO for retirees only would be consistent with the full-service period approach discussed earlier in this chapter. Others take the view that the obligation using a 0 percent cost trend would be consistent with the minimum liability provisions under SFAS No. 87 which do not contain a cost increase factor for future salary increases. The results of this analysis of alternate minimum liability bases for the Field Test companies is presented in table 6.34.

TABLE 6.34 Year Minimum Liability Provisions Become Inoperative under Alternate Liability Bases

Number of companies:	Unfunded APBO for Retirees and Active Eligibles (ED)	Unfunded APBO for Retirees Only	Unfunded Accumulated Obligation with 0% Trend
Year alternate minimum liability provisions inoperative:			
Year 6 and prior	7	17	21
Years 7 — 8	8	5	2
Years 9 — 10	5	2	2
Later than 10 years	6	2	1
	26	26	26

The minimum liability provisions would generally become inoperative earlier under these alternative bases than using the unfunded APBO for retirees and actives fully eligible as proposed in the ED.

Notes

1. In some instances, surviving spouses could not be differentiated from retirees, thus understating the ratio of active employees to retirees.

2. The ARSP is the same for both hypothetical companies because for illustrative purposes, all demographic characteristics other than size were kept the same.

3. The commonly used term "expense" has been used throughout this chapter rather than "net periodic postretirement benefit cost" as defined in the ED.

7

Accounting for Income Taxes

As shown in the previous chapter, a company's expense for retiree health benefits would be higher under accrual accounting than under pay-as-you-go accounting. Moreover, the higher expense under accrual accounting would not generally be deductible under current U.S. federal tax laws because tax deductions for an unfunded plan are currently based on actual benefit payments. Accordingly, to compute the after-tax effect of applying the ED, it is necessary to consider how the difference between the recorded expense and the current tax deduction would be accounted for in computing a company's provision for income taxes.

SFAS No. 96, *Accounting for Income Taxes,* is generally effective starting in 1990 with earlier application encouraged. Accordingly, SFAS No. 96 would be applied in computing a company's income tax provision when the final standard on accounting for postretirement benefits would become effective. This chapter presents an overview of SFAS No. 96 and addresses the specific problems and issues that may arise when accounting for the tax effects under SFAS No. 96 for retiree health benefits. This chapter also presents examples illustrating the necessary computations.

Cautions: The purpose of this chapter is to provide information on how retiree health accruals under the ED might interact with SFAS No. 96. It is not intended to be a comprehensive summary of the many complex provisions in the Statement. Rather, the following discussion is intended to provide some general guidance to those already familiar with the implementation of SFAS No. 96. In addition, the following discussion relates to an unfunded retiree health plan. The impact of SFAS No. 96 on funded plans may differ; companies considering the funding vehicles discussed in chapter 11 should assess the related tax accounting issues. Finally, the discussion and illustrations that follow are based on the provisions of the U.S. federal tax law only. State, local, and foreign jurisdictions with dissimilar tax laws should also be considered.

Overview of SFAS No. 96

A company's provision for income taxes is comprised of the current tax expense plus a provision for the future tax consequences of transactions already recorded in the financial statements ("deferred income taxes"). SFAS No. 96 requires a balance sheet approach (the "liability method") to accounting for deferred income taxes whereby the future tax effect of the difference between the financial statement carrying amount of recorded assets and liabilities and their related tax basis must be measured at each balance sheet date. These differences between a company's book and tax bases of all of its assets and liabilities are referred to as "temporary differences."

Measuring the future tax effects of temporary differences generally requires what is referred to as "scheduling" to determine the future periods in which the tax effects will occur. In other words, it is necessary to determine in what future year or years the temporary differences related to recorded assets or liabilities will "turn around" and be reflected on the tax return. Once all temporary differences have been scheduled, they are totaled by year, resulting in a net taxable or deductible amount for each future period.

Table 7.1 illustrates the calculation of deferred U.S. federal taxes based on a company's temporary differences and their scheduled reversals under SFAS No. 96. This illustration was developed to show how scheduling the reversal of temporary differences and calculating the deferred tax (ignoring the effect of the alternative minimum tax provisions) are generally performed under SFAS No. 96. The statement then requires that deferred taxes be calculated by applying the existing tax law to the net amount of temporary differences reversing in each future year, as if a separate tax return was prepared for each future year. It prohibits assuming future events; in other words, no future income or loss other than that arising from the future tax effect (reversal) of temporary differences which exist at the balance sheet date can be assumed. Therefore, if the reversal of the temporary differences results in a net tax deduction (for example, an excess of expenses recorded for financial accounting purposes, but not yet deductible for tax purposes) in any future year, the tax benefit can be recognized on the financial statements only to the extent that:

- The future deductions can be carried back or forward (on a hypothetical basis in accordance with existing tax law) to offset net taxable amounts (deferred tax credits) occurring in other future periods; or
- The future deduction can be carried back to offset taxes already paid or payable within the carryback period.

TABLE 7.1 Illustration of "Scheduling" of Temporary Differences Under SFAS No. 96

Temporary Difference	Total Amount	1993	1994	1995	1996	1997	1998	1999
Accelerated depreciation	$280	($110)	($110)	$100	$100	$100	$100	$100
Installment sale proceeds	500	250	250	—	—	—	—	—
Retiree health liability*	x	x	x	x	x	x	x	x
Inventory costs capitalized for tax purposes but not for book purposes	(50)	(50)	—	—	—	—	—	—
Litigation accrual	(500)	—	—	—	—	—	—	(500)
	$230	90	140	100	100	100	100	(400)
Carrybacks	—	—	—	—	(100)	(100)	(100)	300
Net taxable (deductible) amounts	$230	90	140	100	—	—	—	(100)**
Tax rates		34%	34%	34%	N/A	N/A	N/A	N/A
Deferred tax liability	$112	$ 31	$ 47	$ 34	$ —	$ —	$ —	$ —

*Future reversal of retiree health temporary difference would be scheduled by year (see remainder of this chapter for discussions of how to determine scheduled amounts).
**Unrecognized net deductible amount

Impact of SFAS No. 96 on Retiree Health Accruals

Because the deferred tax calculations performed under SFAS No. 96 are based on the existing U.S. federal, state, local, or foreign tax laws which often limit the ability to carry over tax losses, the recognition of deferred tax benefits may be limited and the after-tax expense for retiree health benefits under accrual accounting may be higher than would otherwise be expected. To the extent that tax benefits cannot be reflected in income, more of the pretax expense under the ED could fall directly to the "bottom line," directly reducing net income. This can occur in either of two ways:

1. If a company's *total* temporary differences result in a net deductible amount, recognition of this deferred tax debit can occur only to the extent it can be carried back to offset taxes paid or payable within the carryback period (gen-

erally three years under current U.S. federal tax law). Therefore, a company that has significant accrued retiree health liabilities may not have enough offsetting deferred tax credits or taxes previously paid. In this case, any excess net deductible amounts would have no recorded tax benefit and thus could not be recognized in the company's financial statements. (The excess net deductible amounts are commonly referred to as "naked debits.")

2. The future periods in which the retiree health accruals are scheduled to reverse may be such that offsetting deferred tax credit amounts may not be available. For example, this situation could occur if the liability for retiree health benefits was expected to result in tax deductions over a 20-year period, while the other temporary differences were expected to result in taxable amounts over 10 years. In this case, the expected tax deductions for years 11 through 13 may be carried back (for U.S. federal tax purposes) to offset taxable amounts, but amounts in years 14 through 20 could not. This could result in unrecognized tax benefits *even though* the company has a net deferred tax liability on its balance sheet.

In either case, all or a portion of the potential tax benefit related to retiree health accruals would not be recorded in income in the period that the temporary difference arises (e.g., the pretax and after-tax amounts could be the same). Qualifying tax-planning strategies discussed later in this chapter may be available that could mitigate the effects described in 2 above.

Scheduling the Temporary Difference

The reversal of the accrued retiree health liability recorded in the balance sheet must be scheduled by year and included with the company's other temporary differences when computing deferred taxes. To determine how to schedule this temporary difference, it may be appropriate to look to the FASB's guidance for temporary differences related to accrued costs for defined benefit pension plans or deferred compensation contracts.

Caution: The remainder of this chapter discusses some possible approaches for scheduling retiree health temporary differences under SFAS No. 96. Other approaches may also be identified and, ultimately, the FASB may issue specific guidance.

In March 1989, the FASB published its *Special Report* on SFAS No. 96, *A Guide to Implementation of Statement 96 on Accounting for Income Taxes*. Question 12 in the *Special Report* deals with scheduling temporary differences related to

Accounting for Income Taxes 129

pension assets and liabilities. For pension liabilities, a company has the option of consistently following one of two choices (illustrative examples follow):

☐ Approach 1—Schedule reversal based on the amounts by which estimated tax deductions are expected to exceed the interest attributable to the liability for accrued pension cost for the following year and succeeding years, if necessary, until such excess, on a cumulative basis, equals the amount of the temporary difference.

☐ Approach 2—Schedule reversal based on the pattern of present values of estimated tax deductions for the following year and succeeding years, if necessary.

Observation: The Special Report also indicates that if the information necessary to apply either of these approaches would not be available without the enterprise incurring significant incremental actuarial costs on an ongoing basis, the enterprise may schedule reversal ratably over the average remaining service period of employees expected to receive benefits under the plan. However, this exception is rarely expected to be applicable to retiree health benefits, because the actuarial information necessary to apply the scheduling approaches discussed below should generally be available. For this reason, this approach was not illustrated.

Approach 1 is similar to a mortgage loan amortization schedule—"payments" are applied first to "unpaid" interest on the outstanding "loan" balance, and "principal" is reduced only after all interest has been "paid." This approach results in greater interest in early years and more "principal" reductions in later years, just like with a mortgage loan. Applying this theory to the retiree health temporary difference results in greater reversals of the accrued liability in the later years—"back-ending"—because interest on the retiree health obligation generally exceeds the expected tax deduction in the early years and, therefore, no reversal would be scheduled until the later years. This back-end reversal pattern will, in most cases, result in more unrecognized tax benefits than the other approaches discussed below. Accordingly, Approach 1 is not expected to be used in practice.

Approach 2 is based on the "present value approach" for scheduling temporary differences related to assets and liabilities measured at present values (question 10 in the SFAS No. 96 *Special Report*). As compared to Approach 1, the "present value approach" can have the effect of greater scheduled reversals in the early years—front-ending the reversal of the temporary difference. Under this approach, the current present value of each future year's expected tax deduction is the basis for scheduling reversal. For retiree health temporary differences, future tax deductions could generally be based on the stream of present value amounts that, in total, equal the EPBO—or, alternatively, the APBO—as of the end of the year.

Because the EPBO includes the present value of benefits relating to future service, the retiree health liability on the balance sheet—and thus the temporary difference—would never equal the EPBO and, in the early years after transition, the balance sheet liability would generally be only a fraction of the APBO or the EPBO. However, an illustration of the reversal of the temporary difference can be based on the EPBO, using one of two possible approaches—the "ratio" and "first-in, first-out" ("FIFO") methods.

The ratio method is based on the relationship between the balance sheet liability and the EPBO. That ratio is applied to the individual present value amounts that comprise the EPBO in order to determine the scheduled reversals in each year. This method will result in some of the temporary difference being scheduled to reverse in every year a benefit payment is expected to be paid.

The FIFO method is based on the guidance in the *Special Report* that implies a FIFO reversal pattern (i.e., "in the following year and succeeding years, if necessary, until such excess, on a cumulative basis, equals the amount of the temporary difference"). Under the FIFO method, 100 percent of the individual present value amounts comprising the EPBO would be scheduled, starting in the first year and brought forward as many years as necessary to "cover" the amount of the temporary difference.

*Observation: Some believe that an unfunded retiree health plan is analogous to a nonqualified defined benefit pension plan, and would look to the **Special Report** guidance on scheduling temporary differences related to defined benefit pension plans (question 12) in reaching conclusions on how a retiree health temporary difference should be scheduled.*

*Others believe that a retiree health plan is more analagous to unfunded deferred compensation contracts and would look to **Special Report** question 10 (scheduling temporary differences related to assets and liabilities measured at present values) for guidance on scheduling a temporary difference related to an unfunded retiree health plan. Under this analogy, the ratio and FIFO methods of applying the present value approach might be appropriately based on the stream of present values that comprise the APBO (instead of the EPBO). Since the methodology for scheduling is identical whether it is based on the APBO or EPBO, for illustrative purposes only one is shown— based on the EPBO.*

Still others might suggest that a retiree health temporary difference is unique and temporary differences under the FIFO method might be assumed to reverse at amounts equal to the gross value of expected future benefit payments in the following year and in as many subsequent years as necessary. This interpretation would result in a pattern of accelerated reversal that may be advantageous to certain companies in a potential naked debit situation. However, this approach may not be consistent with the guidance in the **Special Report.**

Illustrating the Reversal Pattern

Using the hypothetical highly mature company illustrated in chapter 6, the temporary difference at the end of the year of adoption would be $10.0 million (the $16.2 million accrued expense under the provisions of the ED, less the $6.2 million tax-deductible payments made in the year of adoption) and the EPBO is $126.8 million (the EPBO at the date of transition of $122.0 million rolled forward to the end of the year). Assume further that the actuary has provided the details shown in table 7.2 regarding the EPBO at the end of the year of adoption.

TABLE 7.2 Assumed Pattern of Benefit Payments (in millions)

Year	Gross Amount of Expected Benefit Payments	Present Value of Expected Benefit Payments
1	$6.5	$ 6.2
2	6.9	6.0
3	7.2	5.8
4	7.5	5.5
5	7.8	5.2
6	8.2	5.0
7	8.6	4.8
8	8.9	4.6
9	9.3	4.4
10	9.7	4.2
Thereafter	*	75.1
Total	*	$126.8

* The gross amounts of expected benefit payments after year 10 and in total are not presented because they are not germain to the illustration.

132   Retiree Health Benefits

Using the ratio approach described previously, the $10.0 million temporary difference would be compared with the $126.8 million EPBO. The ratio between those amounts (.0789 in this case) would be applied to *each* of the individual *present value* amounts, by year, that comprise the EPBO. The $10.0 million temporary difference would be scheduled to reverse as shown in table 7.3.

TABLE 7.3   Ratio Approach to Scheduling Temporary Difference (in Millions)

Year	Present Value of Expected Benefit Payments	Ratio	Scheduled Reversals of Temporary Difference**
1	$ 6.2	.0789	$ .49
2	6.0	.0789	.47
3	5.8	.0789	.46
4	5.5	.0789	.44
5	5.2	.0789	.41
6	5.0	.0789	.40
7	4.8	.0789	.38
8	4.6	.0789	.36
9	4.4	.0789	.35
10	4.2	.0789	.33
Thereafter*	75.1	.0789	5.91
Total	$126.8		$10.00

*For illustrative purposes, the reversal schedule has been shown only for the first 10 years, with all subsequent years' reversals combined. In actual practice, it would generally be necessary to schedule the reversal of the temporary difference for more years into the future.

**If the pattern of reversing the retiree health temporary difference had been based on the APBO instead of the EPBO, the scheduled reversals would have been slightly higher in the early years.

Using the FIFO method, the temporary difference would be scheduled to reverse differently depending on whether the gross benefit payments or the present values of the benefits were used. Table 7.4 illustrates the reversal patterns.

TABLE 7.4. Alternate FIFO Approaches to Scheduling Temporary Differences (in Millions)

			Scheduled Reversals of Temporary Difference	
Year	Gross Amount of Expected Benefit Payments	Present Value of Expected Benefit Payments	Based on Gross Payments	Based on Present Values
1	$6.5	$ 6.2	$ 6.5	$ 6.2
2	6.9	6.0	3.5	3.8
3	7.2	5.8	—	—
4	7.5	5.5	—	—
5	7.8	5.2	—	—
6	8.2	5.0	—	—
7	8.6	4.8	—	—
8	8.9	4.6	—	—
9	9.3	4.4	—	—
10	9.7	4.2	—	—
Thereafter	*	75.1		
Total	*	$126.8	$10.0	$10.0

*The gross amounts of expected benefit payments after year 10 and in total are not presented because they are not germain to the illustration.

Tax-Planning Strategies

SFAS No. 96 requires consideration of qualifying tax-planning strategies that could be used, if necessary, to reduce a company's overall deferred tax liability or increase a deferred tax asset. A tax-planning strategy under SFAS No. 96 may be hypothetical, but it must meet both of the following criteria:

- ☐ The strategy must be prudent and feasible, and under management's discretion and control. Management must have both the ability and the intent to implement the strategy, if necessary, to reduce taxes.

- ☐ The strategy cannot involve significant cost to the enterprise—for example, significant expenses to implement the underlying transaction. The potential tax benefit from the strategy cannot be considered when determining whether that strategy gives rise to a significant cost.

SFAS No. 96 prohibits assumptions about future events that are not inherently assumed in the financial statements, such as earning profits in future years.

Future events that *are* inherently assumed in the financial statements are the recovery of assets and the settlement of liabilities *at their reported amounts*. Therefore, a company should assume that the retiree health liability in the balance sheet will be settled at its recorded amount. Thus, tax-planning strategies that change the amount of the underlying liability (e.g., a strategy to amend the plan to reduce or eliminate benefits in the future) would be prohibited under SFAS No. 96.

Observation: As discussed in chapter 11, some funding vehicles that permit current tax deductions are currently available and others may be developed in the future. Although it generally has been difficult to identify qualifying SFAS No. 96 tax-planning strategies that could be used to increase recorded tax benefits related to the settlement of the retiree health liability, more strategies may be available in the future. Generalizations about potential strategies that have been identified (e.g., prefunding benefit payments, subject to the current limitations) are also difficult, because the potential benefit from such a strategy is entirely dependent on the company's other tax attributes. However, the potential choice between the ratio and FIFO scheduling methods previously illustrated may be considered, in a sense, a tax-planning strategy that might allow companies to maximize the recognition of future tax benefits.

8
Effect on Income, Liabilities, and Net Worth

The Field Test included an analysis of the effect that accrual accounting would have on the financial statements of Field Test companies in the initial year of adoption. The Field Test companies' latest financial statements (generally as of December 31, 1988) were obtained, and two scenarios were examined. The first analyzed changes in income, total liabilities, and stockholders' equity using the methodology proposed in the ED, namely prospective recognition of the transition obligation (see chapter 3). The second scenario analyzed the effect of immediate recognition of the transition obligation on income, total liabilities, and stockholders' equity.

Observation: There has been concern by some observers of the FASB project that financial analysts and creditors may, for analytical purposes, deduct the disclosed APBO from the net income or stockholders' equity in the initial year of adoption of accrual accounting, despite the proposed prospective recognition requirement in the ED. Furthermore, some observers of the FASB deliberations have commented that the FASB should permit companies the flexibility to recognize the transition obligation immediately, either as a cumulative catch-up charge against net income or as a direct charge against stockholders' equity. Hence, the Field Test included an analysis of the effect of immediately recognizing the transition obligation.

As indicated in chapter 7, determining a company's after-tax impact of applying accrual accounting is complex. Computing the potential book-tax benefit is difficult under SFAS No. 96, *Accounting for Income Taxes,* and must take into consideration factors beyond the scope of this Field Test, such as the company's other temporary differences.

However, to illustrate the potential impact on net income, liabilities, and net worth, three alternative assumptions were applied to the scenarios described earlier:

- Assumption 1—The higher expense under accrual accounting would be fully tax-effected using a 34 percent effective U.S. federal tax rate. The impact of the effect of state, local, and foreign taxes was ignored.

- Assumption 2—One-half of the higher expense would be tax-effected (34 percent rate); the other half would go directly to reduce net income, dollar-for-dollar.

- Assumption 3—None of the higher expense would be tax-effected but would reduce net income dollar-for-dollar—the so-called "naked debit" situation under SFAS No. 96.

Hypothetical Companies

In order to illustrate the impact of the FASB proposal on income and net worth, pro forma financial statements were developed for the highly mature and immature hypothetical companies presented in chapter 6. Tables 8.2 and 8.3 present the balance sheets and income statements for the hypothetical companies in the year of adoption of accrual accounting. Each table presents the effect of accrual accounting both under the ED and with respect to immediate recognition of the transition obligation for each alternative tax assumption discussed earlier in this chapter. These tables are based on the following information set forth in chapter 6:

	Highly Mature Company	Immature Company
	(Millions)	
Transition obligation (beginning of year)	$98	$23
Accrued expense under the ED for the year (includes approximately $5 million and $1 million of amortization of the transition obligation for the highly mature and immature company, respectively)	16	5
Benefit payments (pay-as-you-go expense)	6	1
Accrued liability (temporary difference)	10	4

Field Test Results

Impact on Pretax Income

Actual operating results for 1988 reported by the Field Test companies were compared to the companies' pretax income (income from continuing operations before the provision for income taxes) after applying the ED. Pretax income was also calculated under the assumption that the transition obligation was immediately recognized (i.e., only current service cost and interest cost would be charged against pretax income). These results are shown in table 8.1.

TABLE 8.1 Impact on Pretax Income—Year of Adoption

	Under ED	Immediate Recognition*
Number of companies with a decrease in pretax income of:		
Less than 2%	2	7
2% — 3.9%	6	5
4% — 7.9%	4	6
8% — 11.9%	3	3
12% — 15.0%	3	0
15.1% — 20%	3	1
Greater than 20%	3	2
Totals	24	24

* Based on an assumption that the transition obligation was charged either to stockholders' equity or directly to net income and thus, the immediate recognition of the obligation does not affect pretax income.

Observation: The impact on income before taxes was dependent on the Field Test companies' operating results for the year. For example, if income levels were unusually high in 1988, the impact of switching to accrual accounting would seem to be lower.

Expense under immediate recognition would be less than that under the ED in the early years after adoption because annual expense would not include amortization of the transition obligation. First year expense under immediate recognition was 14 to 45 percent lower than under the ED for the Field Test companies.

TABLE 8.2 Pro Forma Financial Statements (Year of Adoption)—Highly Mature Hypothetical Company (in Millions)

	As Originally Calculated Under Pay-As-You-Go Accounting	After Applying ED 100% Tax-Effected	After Applying ED 50% Tax-Effected	No Tax Effect
Balance Sheet				
Current assets	$1,000	$1,000	$1,000	$1,000
Noncurrent assets	1,500	1,500	1,500	1,500
Total assets	$2,500	$2,500	$2,500	$2,500
Current liabilities	$ 900	$ 900	$ 900	$ 900
Accrued retiree health liability, net of tax benefit*	—	6	8	10
Long-term debt	700	700	700	700
Total liabilities	1,600	1,606	1,608	1,610
Stockholders' equity	900	894	892	890
Total liabilities and equity	$2,500	$2,500	$2,500	$2,500
Income Statement				
Sales/revenues	$3,000	$3,000	$3,000	$3,000
Accrued retiree health expense*	6	16	16	16
Operating expenses	2,594	2,594	2,594	2,594
Income before taxes	400	390	390	390
Provision for income taxes	150	146	148	150
Income before cumulative catch-up adjustment	250	244	242	240
Cumulative catch-up adjustment	—	—	—	—
Net income	$ 250	$ 244	$ 242	$ 240
Percentage Change				
Long-term debt (including retiree health liability)		0.9%	1.1%	1.4%
Stockholders' equity		0.7	0.9	1.1
Income before taxes		2.5	2.5	2.5
Net income		2.4	3.2	4.0

*Broken out separately and not specifically classified as short- or long-term in the balance sheet for illustrative purposes. In practice, these amounts would not generally be listed separately on the balance sheet and income statement, nor shown net of tax.

Effect on Income, Liabilities, and Net Worth

	Immediate Recognition of Transition Obligation				
Charge to Income			Charge to Stockholders' Equity		
100% Tax-Effected	50% Tax-Effected	No Tax Effect	100% Tax-Effected	50% Tax-Effected	No Tax Effect
$1,000	$1,000	$1,000	$1,000	$1,000	$1,000
1,500	1,500	1,500	1,500	1,500	1,500
$2,500	$2,500	$2,500	$2,500	$2,500	$2,500
$ 900	$ 900	$ 900	$ 900	$ 900	$ 900
68	85	103	68	85	103
700	700	700	700	700	700
1,668	1,685	1,703	1,668	1,685	1,703
832	815	797	832	815	797
$2,500	$2,500	$2,500	$2,500	$2,500	$2,500
$3,000	$3,000	$3,000	$3,000	$3,000	$3,000
11	11	11	11	11	11
2,594	2,594	2,594	2,594	2,594	2,594
395	395	395	395	395	395
148	149	150	148	149	150
247	246	245	247	246	245
65	81	98	—	—	—
$ 182	$ 165	$ 147	$ 247	$ 246	$ 245
9.7%	12.1%	14.7%	9.7%	12.1%	14.7%
7.6	9.4	11.4	7.6	9.4	11.4
1.3	1.3	1.3	1.3	1.3	1.3
27.2	34.0	41.2	1.2	1.6	2.0

TABLE 8.3 Pro Forma Financial Statements (Year of Adoption)—Immature Hypothetical Company (in Millions)

	As Originally Calculated Under Pay-As-You-Go Accounting	After Applying ED 100% Tax-Effected	After Applying ED 50% Tax-Effected	After Applying ED No Tax Effect
Balance Sheet				
Current assets	$ 500	$ 500	$ 500	$ 500
Noncurrent assets	700	700	700	700
Total assets	$1,200	$1,200	$1,200	$1,200
Current liabilities	$ 400	$ 400	$ 400	$ 400
Accrued retiree health liability, net of tax benefit*	—	2	3	4
Long-term debt	700	700	700	700
Total liabilities	1,100	1,102	1,103	1,104
Stockholders' equity	100	98	97	96
Total liabilities and equity	$1,200	$1,200	$1,200	$1,200
Income Statement				
Sales/revenues	$1,000	$1,000	$1,000	$1,000
Accrued retiree health expense*	1	5	5	5
Operating expenses	949	949	949	949
Income before taxes	50	46	46	46
Provision for income taxes	17	15	16	17
Income before cumulative catch-up adjustment	33	31	30	29
Cumulative catch-up adjustment	—	—	—	—
Net income	$ 33	$ 31	$ 30	$ 29
Percentage Change				
Long-term debt (including retiree health liability)		0.3%	0.4%	0.6%
Stockholders' equity		2.0	3.0	4.0
Income before taxes		8.0	8.0	8.0
Net income		6.1	9.1	12.1

*Broken out separately and not specifically classified as short- or long-term in the balance sheet for illustrative purposes. In practice, these amounts would not generally be listed separately on the balance sheet and income statement, nor shown net of tax.

	Immediate Recognition of Transition Obligation				
	Charge to Income			Charge to Stockholders' Equity	
100% Tax-Effected	50% Tax-Effected	No Tax Effect	100% Tax-Effected	50% Tax-Effected	No Tax Effect
$ 500	$ 500	$ 500	$ 500	$ 500	$ 500
700	700	700	700	700	700
$1,200	$1,200	$1,200	$1,200	$1,200	$1,200
$ 400	$ 400	$ 400	$ 400	$ 400	$ 400
16	21	26	16	21	26
700	700	700	700	700	700
1,116	1,121	1,126	1,116	1,121	1,126
84	79	74	84	79	74
$1,200	$1,200	$1,200	$1,200	$1,200	$1,200
$1,000	$1,000	$1,000	$1,000	$1,000	$1,000
4	4	4	4	4	4
949	949	949	949	949	949
47	47	47	47	47	47
15	16	17	15	16	17
32	31	30	32	31	30
15	19	23	—	—	—
$ 17	$ 12	$ 7	$ 32	$ 31	$ 30
2.3%	3.0%	3.7%	2.3%	3.0%	3.7%
16.0	21.0	26.0	16.0	21.0	26.0
6.0	6.0	6.0	6.0	6.0	6.0
48.5	63.6	78.8	3.0	6.1	9.1

Impact on Net Income, Total Liabilities, and Net Worth

As with the impact on pretax income, the impact on net income, total liabilities, and net worth was dependent on the Field Test companies' financial position and not on the relative ratio of active employees to retirees. Using the alternative tax assumptions discussed earlier in this chapter, table 8.4 shows the range of effects of applying the ED to participating Field Test companies' net income, liabilities, and net worth.

TABLE 8.4 Impact of Applying the ED on Net Income, Total Liabilities, and Net Worth — Year of Adoption

	Tax Assumption		
Under the ED	100% Tax-Effected	50% Tax-Effected	No Tax Effect
Number of companies with a decrease in net income of:			
Less than 2%	3	3	2
2% — 4.9%	9	7	7
5% — 9.9%	3	6	5
10% — 19.9%	6	5	5
Greater than 20%	3	3	5
	24	24	24
Number of companies with an increase in total liabilities of:			
Less than 0.5%	9	8	6
0.5% — 1.0%	6	5	7
1.1% — 1.5%	7	7	2
1.6% — 2.0%	1	2	6
Greater than 2%	1	2	3
	24	24	24
Number of companies with a decrease in stockholders' equity of:			
Less than 0.5%	5	3	2
0.5% — 1.0%	6	6	5
1.1% — 1.5%	6	6	2
1.6% — 2.0%	3	2	6
2.1% — 3.0%	2	3	5
Greater than 3%	2	4	4
	24	24	24

Observation: While the prospective transition approach in the ED does mitigate the impact of switching to accrual accounting, for over one-third of the Field Test companies, net income would be reduced by over 10 percent under the ED—even if the temporary difference under SFAS No. 96 is fully tax-effected. Thus, for many companies, the impact on net income could be substantial.

Some may view the above effects on stockholders' equity as relatively minor under the ED with only a few Field Test companies' stockholders' equity decreasing by more than 3 percent. Readers should bear in mind, however, that the Field Test companies are generally financially strong, large, mature or highly mature companies. Thus, it would be improper to assume that these results could be applied to a wider range of companies.

The results in this area were also highly dependent on the tax assumption used (i.e., 100 percent tax-effected, 50 percent tax-effected, or no tax effect). For example, a Field Test company in an assumed naked debit position under SFAS No. 96 (see chapter 7) showed a 16 percent reduction in net income. However, if the temporary difference was fully tax-effected, the reduction in net income would be 10 percent.

Immediate Recognition

If, for analysis purposes, the transition obligation was immediately charged to income as a cumulative catch-up adjustment, net income would decrease significantly in the year of adoption. However, if the transition obligation was charged directly to stockholders' equity, the impact on net income would be relatively minor. In that case, the effect of switching to accrual accounting would generally be the current year's service cost plus interest cost in excess of pay-as-you-go expense. Either way—immediately charging the retiree health obligation to income or equity—will significantly decrease stockholders' equity and increase liabilities. Table 8.5 shows the range of effects of immediate recognition.

Observation: Because the entire transition obligation becomes a temporary difference, the impact of SFAS No. 96 is much more critical when looking at the potential effect of immediate recognition. Thus, for example, a company in a "naked debit" position might have a 26 percent reduction in stockholders' equity, whereas fully tax effecting the temporary difference would result in a 16 percent reduction in equity. As with the other data presented in this chapter, the impact of immediate recognition on the Field Test companies is governed by the general financial strength and profitability of these companies. The impact of the ED on the financial statements of other companies may be of much greater magnitude in the year of adoption.

TABLE 8.5 Impact of Immediate Recognition—Year of Adoption

	Tax Assumption		
	100% Tax-Effected	50% Tax-Effected	No Tax Effect
Immediate Charge to Income (cumulative catch-up adjustment)			
Number of companies with a decrease in net income of:			
Less than 20%	8	7	3
21% — 50%	6	7	8
51% — 100%	7	4	4
101% — 150%	1	4	5
151% — 200%	1	0	1
Greater than 200%	$\frac{1}{24}$	$\frac{2}{24}$	$\frac{3}{24}$
Directly Charging Transition Obligation to Stockholders' Equity			
Number of companies with a decrease in net income of:			
Less than 2%	10	7	4
2% — 5%	6	9	11
6% — 10%	6	5	3
Greater than 10%	$\frac{2}{24}$	$\frac{3}{24}$	$\frac{6}{24}$
Immediate Recognition—Cumulative Catch-up Against Income or Direct Charge to Stockholders' Equity			
Number of companies with an increase in total liabilities:			
Less than 3%	8	6	5
3.0% — 5.0%	4	3	3
5.1% — 10.0%	7	5	5
10.1% — 15.0%	4	6	6
15.1% — 20.0%	1	3	4
Greater than 20%	$\frac{0}{24}$	$\frac{1}{24}$	$\frac{1}{24}$
Number of companies with a decrease in stockholders' equity:			
Less than 5%	6	5	5
5.0% — 10%	5	5	4
10.1% — 15%	6	3	2
15.1% — 20%	3	5	4
20.1% — 30%	3	4	5
Greater than 30%	$\frac{1}{24}$	$\frac{2}{24}$	$\frac{4}{24}$

Debt/Equity Ratio

Since application of the ED affects liabilities and stockholders' equity, a company's debt-to-equity ratio will be affected to some degree. The magnitude of the effect depends on the increased expense under accrual accounting and the related tax effect computed under SFAS No. 96. Immediate recognition of the transition obligation, of course, would have the greatest impact on a company's debt/equity ratio.

Caution: It should be noted that financial analysts, creditors, rate makers, and regulatory agencies probably will have different concepts as to the method of evaluating a company's financial position after applying the ED.

Observation: In general, the impact of the ED on the debt-to-equity ratio will depend on the size and financial strength of the company. The size of the company should be considered because both the numerator and denominator of the ratio calculation is affected by the accrual of retiree health liabilities (increasing recorded liabilities while decreasing stockholders' equity). Thus, the debt-to-equity ratios of smaller companies may be changed to a greater extent than those of larger companies.

Conclusion

As shown above, the overall financial statement impact in the year of adoption is heavily dependent on the transition approach. Immediate recognition of the transition obligation could significantly reduce stockholders' equity and a company's debt-to-equity ratio. The impact of prospective transition, following the ED approach, will be less drastic, but still very significant. In either case, the effect of computing the related tax benefit under SFAS No. 96 will be important for companies to consider when evaluating the impact of the ED.

Caution: The results on income and net worth for the Field Test companies may not be representative of companies in general. In addition, in some cases, not all of a company's retiree health plans were included in the Field Test. Also, the companies' other postretirement benefit plans (e.g., retiree life insurance) that were not included in the Field Test may be significant. Therefore, the overall impact of the ED on the participating companies' income, total liabilities, and net worth may be understated.

9
The Impact of Medicare Catastrophic Coverage

The Medicare Catastrophic Coverage Act (the Act) was signed into law on July 1, 1988. The Act is intended to protect Medicare beneficiaries from catastrophic medical expenses, including hospital, physician, and prescription drug bills. The Act increases the amounts and kinds of health care Medicare will pay for, thereby reducing many companies' costs for retiree health benefits.

The provisions of the new law are phased in over a four-year period beginning on January 1, 1989. Table 9.2 provides a comparison of prior law with the expanded Medicare coverage.

Since the Act was not effective on the January 1, 1988 Field Test valuation date, its provisions were not taken into account for purposes of the valuations. However, as part of the Field Test, a special analysis was performed to provide additional information on the impact of Medicare catastrophic coverage. This chapter summarizes the Act and its impact on obligations and expense as of the January 1, 1988 valuation date.

The Act

In the largest expansion of Medicare since 1965, the Act adds several new features to the program, including:

- ☐ payment for unlimited inpatient hospitalization (Medicare Part A) after payment of an annual deductible (effective in 1989);

- ☐ an outpatient prescription drug benefit (subject to coinsurance—phased in from 1991 to 1993) after payment of an annual deductible ($550 in 1990, rising to $652 in 1992 and indexed thereafter);

- a limit on out-of-pocket expenses for physician and certain other Part B services starting at $1,370 (effective in 1990) and;
- increased Part B premiums and an additional surtax based on income tax liability for financing the benefits.

Medicare Part A

Prior to the Act, Medicare Part A (which is financed through hospital insurance payroll taxes) covered certain inpatient hospital services, skilled nursing facilities, home health care, hospice care, and blood products for most individuals age 65 and over and disabled individuals. Benefits were provided and deductibles and coinsurance provisions were required generally with reference to each "spell of illness."

The Act modified these Part A provisions, expanded coverage for certain inpatient benefits, and eliminated the spell of illness concept.

Inpatient Hospital Services

As of January 1, 1989, Medicare will cover an unlimited number of days of inpatient hospital services covered under Part A (excluding psychiatric care) after the beneficiary pays a calendar year deductible (estimated to be $564 in 1989). Thus, the prior inpatient hospital deductible and Part A coinsurance will no longer be applied to each spell of illness, and the Medicare limit on the number of covered inpatient hospital days (90 days of inpatient care per spell of illness plus 60 lifetime reserve days) is eliminated.

Observation: By limiting beneficiary out-of-pocket expenses for inpatient hospitalization to one annual deductible and eliminating Part A coinsurance, many of the costs of extensive or repeated hospitalization associated with catastrophic illness will now be paid for by Medicare.

Medicare Part B

Part B coverage includes physicians' and certain other practitioners' services, outpatient hospital services, additional home health visits, and other medical and health services not covered under Part A. Part B requires beneficiaries to pay premiums to participate in Part B (some employers pay all or part of the Part B premiums).

Out-of-Pocket Maximum

Beginning in 1990, an annual out-of-pocket limit (starting at $1,370) on a beneficiary's Part B deductible and coinsurance of Medicare-allowable charges will be added to the Medicare program. Expenses for the annual $75 Part B deductible, the blood deductible, and Part B 20 percent coinsurance of Medicare-allowable charges will go towards satisfying the annual limit. Once the out-of-pocket maximum is reached, Medicare will be required to pay for 100 percent of the Medicare-allowable costs or charges for any additional Part B covered services for the beneficiary.

Observation: *Since Medicare may not pay all provider charges, individuals or employers may still have to pay amounts over Medicare-allowable charges.*

The out-of-pocket maximum is to be indexed for future years so that a constant proportion of Medicare beneficiaries (7 percent according to Congressional Budget Office estimates) would meet or exceed the catastrophic limit each year.

Home Health Services

Medicare will pay for an increased number of days for covered home nursing care and home health aide services furnished on or after January 1, 1990.

New Part B Benefits

Outpatient prescription drugs. Currently, Medicare does not offer an outpatient prescription drug benefit. However, by January 1, 1991, Medicare will pay for all Medicare-covered outpatient prescription drugs, subject to a large deductible and coinsurance requirement. The drug deductible (completely separate from the Part B deductible) is set at $600 for 1991, $652 for 1992, and will be indexed for future years. Outpatient drugs will be subject to 50 percent coinsurance in 1991, 40 percent in 1992, and 20 percent thereafter. These coinsurance amounts will not be applied to the Part B out-of-pocket maximum.

To receive payment for outpatient drugs, Medicare beneficiaries will be required to provide satisfactory proof of expenses during the year over the deductible amount. In addition, a procedure is established to limit the amount Medicare will pay for each covered outpatient prescription.

Other Part B benefits. Beginning January 1, 1990, Medicare coverage is expanded for home intravenous (I-V) therapy drugs and associated services, mammography screening, and respite care.

Financing of Benefits

The Medicare Part A and Part B catastrophic benefits are to be financed through the combination of an additional flat Part B premium and a supplemental premium (surtax) based on income tax liability.

Additional Part B premium. The Act provides for increases to the existing monthly Part B premium ($27.90 in 1989) to finance the new catastrophic illness and prescription drug benefits. In 1989, a flat premium increase of $4.00 per month is added to the Part B premium; this additional premium is to rise to $10.20 per month in 1993. The additional Part B premium will be indexed for future years. A beneficiary's Social Security benefit will not be reduced below the current level despite an increase in the additional Part B premium.

Observation: Those employers who now pay the Part B premium should carefully consider whether, and to what extent, they will pay the additional Part B premium.

Additional surtax. An additional income tax-related surtax will be imposed on certain Medicare beneficiaries. Under the Act, individuals eligible for Part A for more than six months during the taxable year and having $150 or more of federal income tax liability must pay a new income tax-related surtax. The rate in 1989 is $22.50 per $150 of adjusted federal income tax liability, and would rise to $42.00 per $150 of adjusted federal income tax liability in 1993.

The maximum surtax per beneficiary for 1989 is $800. This maximum will increase to $1,050 in 1993 and will be indexed thereafter. The maximum surtax for a married couple filing a joint tax return where both individuals are enrolled in Medicare is twice the amount for a single beneficiary ($1,600 in 1989).

In the case of a married couple with only one spouse enrolled in Medicare, the surtax would be computed on the basis of half the joint tax liability of the couple.

Observation: Some recent estimates show that the surtax may generate revenues greater than what is needed to fund the benefits. Congressional hearings are planned to investigate the issue to determine whether the surtax should be reduced.

Maintenance of Effort

The Act contains a "maintenance of effort" provision under which most companies providing retiree health benefits are required to give additional benefits or cash refunds equal to the benefits now duplicated under Medicare. Companies that, as of July 1, 1988, provided health benefits that duplicated 50 percent or more of the actuarial value of the new Medicare benefits are required to either increase benefits or pay eligible retirees (and, according to the Health Care Financing Administration (HCFA), their dependents if eligible for Medicare benefits) the cash value of the benefits that will now be paid by Medicare. Companies are required to rebate the duplicative Part A benefits in 1989 and Part B benefits in 1990.

In December 1988, HCFA issued a Notice announcing the national average actuarial value of duplicative Part A benefits so that companies may comply with the 1989 part of the maintenance of effort provision. The national actuarial value of Medicare Part B benefits is scheduled to be published by HCFA before January 1990.

In computing the actuarial value of the duplicative Part A benefits in 1989, companies have the option of using the national average actuarial values established by HCFA, or calculating the value based on the guidelines provided by HCFA in its Notice, and following generally accepted actuarial practices.

HCFA determined that the national average actuarial value of the duplicative Part A benefits now provided by Medicare was $61 per capita as of July 1, 1988 (the date employers must use to determine if their benefits meet the 50 percent test).

Therefore, any company that provided duplicative Part A benefits worth at least $30.50 as of July 1, 1988, must comply with the maintenance of effort provision in 1989. It is anticipated that most employers providing retiree health benefits will meet this 50 percent test and will have to comply with the maintenance of effort provision.

Those companies that meet this test will then have to determine the amount (in benefits, cash, or a combination of both) that must be refunded to retirees. For purposes of the refund, HCFA has determined the 1989 national average actuarial value of Part A benefits to be $65 per capita. Therefore, companies meeting the 50 percent test will have to provide additional benefits or cash refunds equal to $65 per capita unless it can be demonstrated, based on a company's own experience, that the value of duplicative Part A benefits is less than $65 per capita. The Notice specifically allows employers to determine their own costs following generally accepted actuarial practices.

Observation: It appears that $65 may be greater than the value of duplicative Part A benefits provided by many companies. This depends, of course, on the specific provisions of the company's plan and the health benefit utilization *patterns of their retiree group. Some companies will therefore find it beneficial to determine the actuarial value of the duplicative Part A benefits based on their own experience.*

The HCFA Notice also provides the following guidance:

- any cash refund of Part A duplicative benefits must be made before the end of 1989;
- a company can satisfy the maintenance of effort provision by making all or a part of the refund in the form of an offset against current employee premiums or a planned premium rate increase (provided the increase was planned and communicated prior to July 1, 1988);
- employers do not have to comply with the maintenance of effort provision with respect to individuals for whom Medicare is the secondary payer; and
- special rules apply for employers that contract with HMOs on a risk basis.

The Effects of the Medicare Catastrophic Coverage Act

To provide additional information to the Field Test companies, a methodology was developed to estimate the effects of the Medicare Catastrophic Coverage Act on their obligations and expense as of the January 1, 1988 valuation date. (A description of the methodology is provided later in this chapter.)

To illustrate the impact of the Act, table 9.1 shows the percent savings (rounded to the nearest percent) in the components of projected obligations (the APBO and EPBO) and 1988 expense under the ED due to Medicare catastrophic coverage for two sample Field Test companies. Both companies used the carve-out method to integrate payments with Medicare.

TABLE 9.1 Percent Change Due to Medicare Catastrophic Coverage—As of January 1, 1988

	Company P	Company Q
APBO		
Retirees	(11%)	(25%)
Actives fully eligible	(14)	(21)
Actives not yet fully eligible	(5)	(14)
Total APBO	(6)	(20)
EPBO	(5)	(18)
1988 expense under ED	(5)	(19)

The analysis of the impact of Medicare catastrophic coverage on the Field Test companies shows a general reduction in first year expense under the ED ranging from less than 2 percent to nearly 24 percent (using an assumption that 75 percent of submitted charges for Part B services were Medicare-allowable). For some companies, a sensitivity analysis was performed assuming that all (100 percent) submitted charges for Part B services were Medicare-allowable and thus, Medicare would pay for all submitted charges over the out-of-pocket limit. This sensitivity analysis yielded reductions in first year expense under the ED ranging from 7 percent to slightly over 25 percent. It is also interesting to note that, for many of the Field Test companies, the percentage reduction in APBO was very close to the percentage reduction in first year expense.

Observation: The reductions in expense under the ED due to Medicare catastrophic coverage depends on many factors, including demographics (e.g., the ratio of actives to retirees and distribution of retirees between those under 65 and those 65 and over), utilization, the method used to integrate payments with Medicare, and the assumptions used.

Methodology

For purposes of estimating the impact of Medicare catastrophic coverage on the obligations and 1988 expense of the Field Test companies, the entire Act was assumed to be in effect as of January 1, 1988, rather than being phased in over a four-year period. In general, claims for each individual were recalculated as if Medicare would pay amounts in excess of the new catastrophic limits, expressed in dollar amounts for the experience period (generally 1986). Appropriate deductible and coinsurance amounts were then applied. Several of the Field Test companies were unable to provide the data needed to make this estimate.

Inpatient Hospital

Medicare will now pay for all Part A covered services after payment of one annual deductible rather than a per admission deductible. The actual 1986 Part A deductible was $492. Therefore, all inpatient hospital claims that were greater than this amount for the experience period were captured by individual, and the percentage savings determined was used as an estimate of the likely percentage savings in the future.

Drugs

The Medicare Catastrophic Coverage Act provides for payment of all covered prescription drugs after a $652 deductible in 1992, subject to coinsurance. For this analysis, the deductible was stated as a dollar value for the experience period. Where possible, all eligible drug claims for an individual in excess of this amount were captured and assumed to be paid by Medicare. For most of the companies it was not possible to distinguish between those drugs that will be covered by Medicare and those that will be excluded. For example, certain "experimental" drugs will not be covered by Medicare. However, this should not significantly affect the estimate.

Part B

The maximum Part B out-of-pocket limit of $1,370 was expressed in a dollar value for the experience period. The effect of this maximum was estimated by capturing all claims (on a person-by-person basis) in excess of this amount for Part B type services.

Estimates of the percent Medicare will pay for in the future were computed assuming that only 75 percent of submitted charges were allowable by Medicare. Disallowed charges were not counted toward the Part B out-of-pocket limit. It was assumed that Medicare would cover 75 percent of the submitted charges after the individual had incurred Medicare-allowable charges for the year equal to the Part B out-of-pocket limit for the experience period. The remaining 25 percent would be paid by the company.

In some cases, a sensitivity analysis was performed assuming 100 percent of submitted charges were Medicare-allowable. Therefore, all charges in excess of the Part B out-of-pocket limit for the experience period were assumed to be covered by Medicare.

The difficulty of estimating Part B savings. Medicare-allowable charges are claim amounts for Part B services that are eligible for payment by Medicare. Allowable charges are limited to certain types of services and certain dollar amounts for those covered services. Medicare only pays 80 percent of allowable charges. Employers often cover both the 20 percent not covered by Medicare as well as those charges that exceed the allowable limit. Because of the difficulty in determining Medicare-allowable charges, estimates of Part B savings are subject to a greater degree of variation than the Part A and drug categories.

Estimates of Part B savings are further complicated by the fact that physician charge patterns vary in different parts of the country. For example, in certain states, 80 percent of all physicians accept Medicare payment as full payment (the individual patient does not owe the doctor any fees over-and-above the Medicare-allowable charge for covered services). In other states, however, as few as 20 percent of all doctors accept Medicare as full payment for covered services. This variation contributes to the difficulty of determining the impact of Medicare catastrophic coverage on Part B costs.

TABLE 9.2 Prior Law and New Law Comparison of Medicare Part A and Part B

	Prior Law	New Law*
Medicare Part A		
Inpatient Hospital Services		
☐ Deductible ($540 in 1988; estimated $564 in 1989)	One per spell of illness	One per calendar year (if deductible paid in December, no additional deductible for hospitalization beginning January of following year)
☐ Covered inpatient days	90 days per spell of illness, plus 60-day lifetime reserve	No day limitation for acute care (except psychiatric care)
☐ Coinsurance	One-fourth of the inpatient deductible per day for days 61-90 per spell of illness, plus one-half of the inpatient deductible per day for lifetime reserve days	No coinsurance requirement
☐ Blood deductible	Three pints per spell of illness	Three pints per calendar year
Inpatient Psychiatric Care		
☐ Deductible	Inpatient hospital deductible applies	Inpatient hospital deductible applies
☐ Covered inpatient days	190 per lifetime	190 per lifetime
☐ Coinsurance	Inpatient hospital coinsurance applies	No coinsurance requirement
☐ Hospitalized on Medicare eligibility date	Covered days reduced for hospitalizations during the 150 days prior to eligibility	Covered days reduced for hospitalizations during the 150 days prior to eligibility and restriction applies until out of hospital for 60 consecutive days
Skilled Nursing Facilities		
☐ Covered days	100 days per spell of illness	150 days per calendar year

* Unless otherwise specified, all benefits effective January 1, 1989.

TABLE 9.2 Prior Law and New Law Comparison of Medicare Part A and Part B (continued)

	Prior Law	New Law*
☐ Coinsurance	Nothing for first 20 days per spell of illness; one-eighth of inpatient hospital deductible per day for days 21-100 per spell of illness	20% of national average Medicare per diem skilled nursing facility rate (approximately $20.50 in 1989) for first 8 days during the calendar year
☐ Prior hospitalization	Must have 3 days prior hospitalization	Prior hospitalization not required
Hospice Care		
☐ Covered days	Two 90-day periods and one 30-day period	No maximum if the attending physician or hospice medical director recertifies the beneficiary as terminally ill
☐ Coinsurance	None (except for respite care and outpatient drugs)	None (except for respite care and outpatient drugs)
Home Health Care		
☐ Deductible	None	None
☐ Coinsurance	None	None
☐ Daily coverage	Intermittent skilled nursing care visits for up to 5 days a week for up to two or three weeks	Effective 1/1/90, nursing care and home health aides can be provided 7 days a week for up to 38 consecutive days
Medicare Part B		
Deductible	$75 per calendar year	$75 per calendar year
Coinsurance	20% of Medicare-allowable charges above the deductible amount (50% for outpatient psychiatric services)	20% of Medicare-allowable charges above the deductible amount up to out-of-pocket maximum (50% for psychiatric services); 0% of Medicare-allowable charges above out-of-pocket maximum

TABLE 9.2 Prior Law and New Law Comparison of Medicare Part A and Part B (continued)

	Prior Law	New Law*
Out-of-Pocket Maximum		
☐ Annual limit	None	$1370 in 1990; indexed for future years
☐ Payment over limit	Not applicable	100% of Medicare-allowable charges for covered Part B services incurred during remainder of calendar year
☐ Expenses counting toward limit	Not applicable	Part B deductible, blood deductible (three pints per calendar year), and coinsurance
Outpatient Prescription Drugs		
☐ Covered drugs	Limited to immunosuppressive drugs furnished within one year of an organ transplant	Beginning 1/1/90, home I-V therapy drugs (initially antibiotics only) and immunosuppresive drugs (without prior limit); effective 1/1/91, all other outpatient drugs marketed prior to 1938 or approved by Food and Drug Administration
☐ Deductible	Generally not applicable	$550 in 1990, $600 in 1991, and $652 in 1992; after 1992 deductible indexed so that approximately 17% of beneficiaries would exceed deductible
☐ Coinsurance	Generally not applicable	20% for I-V drugs, 50% for immunosuppressives; for all others: 50% in 1991, 40% in 1992, and 20% thereafter
☐ Prescription day limit	Not applicable	Prescriptions generally limited to a 30-day supply

TABLE 9.2 Prior Law and New Law Comparison of Medicare Part A and Part B (continued)

	Prior Law	New Law*
Home I-V Drug Services		
☐ Covered services	None	Beginning 1/1/90, supplies, equipment, nursing, and pharmacy services associated with home I-V drug therapy prescribed by physician
☐ Deductible	Not applicable	None
☐ Coinsurance	Not applicable	None
Mammography Screenings		
☐ Eligibility	Generally not available	Effective 1/1/90, available every other year for women 65 and older; for disabled women under 65, available on increasing basis, up to one per year
☐ Benefit	None	Subject to 20% coinsurance on lower of actual charge, fee schedule allowance, or reasonable charge limit ($50 in 1990)
Respite Care		
☐ Covered services	Only available as a part of hospice care	Effective 1/1/90, services of homemaker, home health aide, personal care services, licensed nursing care to chronically dependent individuals whose Part B expenses exceed the out-of-pocket maximum or whose prescription drug expenses exceed the prescription drug deductible
☐ Length of coverage	Generally not applicable	Up to 80 hours per calendar year

TABLE 9.2 Prior Law and New Law Comparison of Medicare Part A and Part B (continued)

	Prior Law	New Law*
☐ Coinsurance	Generally not applicable	20% coinsurance applies regardless of whether Part B limit met
Outpatient Mental Health		
☐ Coverage	Limited to 50% of cost, up to $250 per calendar year	Limited to 50% of cost, up to $250 per calendar year
Maintenance of Effort		
☐ Affected employers	None	Employers who currently provide benefits that duplicate at least 50% of the actuarial value of the new Part A and B benefits (excluding covered outpatient drugs)
☐ Determination of benefits	Not applicable	Actuarial value of duplicative benefits based on national average values or the employer's own actuarial values (net of employee premiums)
☐ Effective date	Not applicable	Part A benefits in 1989 (only), Part B benefits in 1990 (only)—or expiration of collective bargaining agreement, if later
Premiums		
☐ Part A	Payroll tax on workers covered under Old Age, Survivors, and Disability Insurance program (OASDI)	Payroll tax on workers covered under OASDI

TABLE 9.2 Prior Law and New Law Comparison of Medicare Part A and Part B (continued)

	Prior Law	New Law*
☐ Part B	Basic Part B premium: $27.90 per month (1989); indexed for future years	Basic Part B premium plus flat monthly premium: $4.00 in 1989, $4.90 in 1990, $7.40 in 1991, $9.20 in 1992, $10.20 in 1993, indexed for future years
☐ Supplemental premium	None	Required by individuals eligible for Part A benefits; rates per $150 of adjusted federal income tax liability: $22.50 in 1989, $37.50 in 1990, $39.00 in 1991, $40.50 in 1992, $42.00 in 1993, indexed for future years Annual maximums established

10
Strategies for Cost Management and Plan Design

Prompted by the escalating cost of retiree health plans and the proposed change in accounting for these benefits, the Field Test companies and others are looking for ways to better manage and control the costs of these plans. As a result, many companies are now developing strategies for short- and long-term cost management and plan design. These strategies often involve flexibility and periodic re-evaluations—to respond to changes in corporate priorities, retiree needs, utilization or demographic changes, the health care environment, or the government's role in providing health care.

In addressing short-term concerns, it is essential to first understand the current costs of the benefits program and the possible impact of the FASB's Exposure Draft. The next goal would be to look for better ways to manage and control future costs while still providing a competitive compensation and benefits package.

An important early step in this process generally involves an analysis of a company's benefits philosophy and its overall retiree income program—including pensions, savings plans, spousal benefits, Social Security, and other sources of income—realizing that health benefits are only part of a larger package. Retirees may depend on these other sources of income to pay health care costs, such as their required contributions, deductibles, and coinsurance. Careful review of early retirement incentives may also be appropriate, since retirees under age 65 are generally not eligible for Medicare, resulting in greater employer costs. In addition, some retirees may have other employers providing health benefits, and it is appropriate to consider how these benefits are coordinated with Medicare and other coinsurers.

Once benefit objectives are clear and current plan design has been analyzed, it should prove easier for management to consider various cost control techniques. However, to develop and implement effective strategies often requires a high-level task force of financial, human resources, and legal management.

This chapter first discusses some of the plan design options available to companies as they develop cost management strategies. A brief overview of constraints that often must be considered in analyzing plan design options follows. The chapter concludes with a discussion of selected long-term considerations affecting cost management.

Plan Design Options

Although there are no simple solutions to the complex problem of controlling retiree health costs while maintaining acceptable quality care, some benefit design alternatives can be effective. Benefit design changes fall into three broad categories: cost sharing, changing the nature of benefits, and managed care. Some companies may implement only one type of design change, such as increasing retiree contributions, while others may decide to implement several together, in a comprehensive benefit restructuring.

Cost-Sharing Strategies

Cost sharing—requiring retirees and dependents to share the cost of their health care—clearly has been an increasingly important feature of retiree health plan design. Cost sharing permits an employer to offer the same benefits, but shifts some costs to retirees.

Many of the cost-sharing techniques used by companies to reduce health care costs for active employees—e.g., increased deductibles, copayments, annual or lifetime maximum benefits, and employee (retiree) contributions—may help to reduce a company's retiree health costs. Increased cost sharing may also encourage retirees and their dependents to be more cost effective in their use of health care services, thus possibly reducing the level of future cost increases.

Table 10.1 summarizes popular cost-sharing strategies and provides some practical observations.

Medicare Integration
Another technique of cost sharing involves the manner in which the employer's retiree health plan integrates or coordinates with Medicare.

- In a typical *coordination of benefits* (COB) plan, up to 100 percent of a retiree's total covered expenses will be paid, with Medicare payments first

TABLE 10.1 Selected Cost-Sharing Strategies

Cost-Sharing Strategy	Observation
Index deductibles, copayments, out-of-pocket maximums or retiree contributions; index to increases in plan's claims experience or medical care component of CPI.	☐ Helps to control company costs. ☐ Retirees assume some economic risk. ☐ Partially eliminates impact of health inflation on future company costs and can maintain ratio of retiree to company share of costs. ☐ If included in terms of plan, would be anticipated in projecting obligations and expense under the ED.
Non-indexed deductibles, copayments, out-of-pocket maximums or retiree contributions.	☐ Gives company flexibility to increase on an ad hoc basis. ☐ When ad hoc increases made, treated as plan amendments under the ED.
Non-indexed lifetime or annual benefit maximums.	☐ Will cap company costs at maximum. ☐ Any increases would be treated as plan amendments under the ED when made (unless present "substantive commitment" to increase caps).
Base cost sharing on years of service.	☐ Reduces cost for employees with less service and provides greater benefits for longer service employees. ☐ Depending on specific design, may accrue costs under ED to expected retirement age. ☐ Encourages longer service. ☐ If retiree contributions automatically indexed, there may be reduced obligation and expense under ED.
Base cost sharing on annual pay at retirement or pension income.	☐ Higher paid employees have greater cost sharing. ☐ Reduces expense and obligations.

applied to reduce the retiree's obligation under the plan and remaining Medicare payments (if any) applied to reduce the company's obligation.

- ☐ In a *Medicare exclusion* arrangement, the plan benefit is based on the net amount of covered expenses after the Medicare payment is applied.
- ☐ In a *Medicare carve-out* arrangement, Medicare payments are first applied to reduce benefits otherwise payable by the company.

These methods are illustrated in table 10.2, which is based on a plan with a $100 deductible and 20 percent coinsurance, and $1,000 of covered claims, with a $700 Medicare payment. Table 10.2 also illustrates the various costs for a retiree under age 65.

TABLE 10.2 Medicare Integration

	(a) Pre-Medicare	(b) COB	(c) Exclusion	(d) Carve-Out
Covered claims	$1,000	$1,000	$1,000	$1,000
Medicare payment	0	700	700	700
Company payment	720	300	160	20
Retiree payment	280	0	140	280

(a) Without Medicare (or for a retiree under age 65), the retiree would pay a $100 deductible plus 20% of the remaining $900, or $180, for a total of $280. The company would be responsible for the remaining $720.

(b) Under a *COB arrangement,* the $700 Medicare payment would first be applied to reduce the retiree's $280 obligation to zero. The $420 of remaining Medicare payments would then be applied to reduce the company's obligation from $720 to $300.

(c) If the plan used the *exclusion method* of Medicare integration, Medicare would pay $700 of the $1,000 of covered expenses, leaving $300 of expenses. The retiree would pay a $100 deductible plus 20% of the remaining $200, or $40, for a total of $140. The company would then be responsible for the remaining $160 ($300-$140).

(d) If the plan integrated with Medicare under the *carve-out method,* the $700 Medicare payment would be fully applied to reduce the company's $720 obligation to $20. The retiree's obligation would be $280, unreduced by Medicare payments.

As can be seen in table 10.2, COB is the most costly method of Medicare integration for a company and carve-out is the least costly method. Changing the method by which retiree benefits are integrated with Medicare payments may reduce the proportion of retiree health costs paid by the company.

Changes in Nature of Company Benefit Plans

This section describes various techniques that involve changing the nature of the company's benefit plans.

Gear Eligibility and/or Benefits to Length of Service

Eligibility for full benefits is often based on a minimum of years of service and attainment of a specific age, or the sum of age plus service (e.g., full benefits if the sum of age plus service equals or exceeds 75).

By imposing eligibility requirements that are related to longer periods of service, companies can encourage and reward longer service employees. At the same time, costs are reduced as shorter service employees receive nothing or less than full company-paid benefits. Similarly, the eligibility for costly spousal benefits would be tightened.

Some companies are considering changing the duration of benefits by providing retiree health benefits for a period equal to the length of service (e.g., a retiree with 10 years of service would receive retiree health benefits for 10 years). This technique obviously rewards longer service and limits costs for shorter service employees.

An important consideration in a length of service formula is the effect of the Internal Revenue Code Section 89 nondiscrimination rules (see discussion later in this chapter).

Scheduled Benefits Plan

In a scheduled benefits plan, company-paid benefits are restricted to paying certain amounts for particular health services or products, regardless of the actual cost. The company may determine its own reimbursement levels for hospital and physician care, or may use reimbursement levels developed by others, such as using Medicare diagnostic related groups (DRGs) for retirees under age 65. For example, the plan could pay $15 for every covered doctor's visit and $30 for every x-ray, regardless of the actual cost. A scheduled benefits plan limits the amount a company must pay for each health-related product or service, but does not set a limit on the overall cost, which will be determined by the volume of health care used.

Table 10.3 shows some advantages and disadvantages of a scheduled benefits plan.

Dollar-Denominated Benefits

A company can change the nature of its financial commitment to its benefits plan by providing a determined dollar amount toward the cost of retiree health benefits, instead of an open-ended commitment to pay for health care benefits regardless of cost.

TABLE 10.3 Scheduled Benefits Plan

Advantages	Disadvantages
☐ Retirees may be more cost conscious in obtaining health care.	☐ If indexed to inflation, company bears increases.
☐ Can be tied into Medicare reimbursement levels (including Medicare catastrophic coverage).	☐ Difficult to communicate.
	☐ May be difficult and costly to administer.
☐ Company obligation for future inflation can be predicted or controlled.	
☐ Ad hoc increases treated as plan amendments under ED.	

In a dollar-denominated benefits plan, each retiree receives a fixed annual amount to be used to pay for health benefits at retirement. For example, retirees under age 65 could receive $2,500 per year for family coverage, and retirees age 65 and over could receive $750 per year. The retiree generally must pay the costs of coverage exceeding the amounts provided by the company and not paid for by Medicare. Dollar-denominated benefits can be varied by age at retirement, length of service, number of dependents, or Medicare eligibility.

The company may retain discretion as to when and how to increase the dollar amount or may include automatic increases for inflation. This flexibility permits a company to reduce its costs while gradually transferring responsibility for payment of health care costs to retirees. The plan must, of course, be carefully structured, since retirees generally assume those costs exceeding the company's contribution.

Under the ED, a company's expense and obligation under this type of plan are generally limited, since the dollar-denominated amount is fixed and no health care cost trend assumption would be required. Of course, increases in the dollar-denominated benefits should be very carefully planned, taking into account projected costs, since ad hoc increases will be treated as plan amendments, and could have a significant impact under the ED.

As discussed later, however, there are a number of constraints to consider in changing the benefit to a dollar-denominated program.

Multiple Options and Flexible Benefits

A company may offer retirees different health plan options with various levels of benefits in exchange for higher or lower retiree cost sharing. For example, a company may offer retirees a choice of an employer-pay-all plan with an annual deductible of $500, or a plan where the retiree makes a monthly contribution to lower the annual deductible to $100.

These types of plans can be simple, multiple option arrangements, or complex flexible benefit programs. A flexible benefit program for retirees can provide each retiree with a certain amount of "benefit credits" each year, depending on his length of service with the company. These benefit credits may be used by the retiree to purchase life, dental, and health insurance from among several options. Each year, the company determines the number of credits it will award per year of service, in an effort to predict and control its future obligations. If the retiree does not have enough benefit credits to purchase the desired insurance, he may pay the difference on an after-tax basis. Flexible benefits offer retirees the opportunity to select the most meaningful benefits for themselves, and may serve to limit the company's commitment. Accounting for a flexible benefit arrangement depends on how the plan is structured.

Cash or Other Benefits

Offering active eligible and retired employees cash or other compensation in lieu of health benefits may produce cost savings over the long term. For example, requiring retirees to purchase coverage on their own and providing periodic cash payments to apply toward their health insurance premium expense can result in considerable company savings. However, it may be unacceptable to switch retirees into costly individual health coverage. Some companies are considering offering voluntary programs whereby retirees may opt out of participation in the health plan in exchange for a lump-sum payment.

Observation: *This type of lump sum "cash out" may be treated as a settlement of the postretirement benefit obligation under the ED. However, such a program would require the employer to make a large cash commitment and does not assure that retirees would use these funds for health care.*

Other companies may offer retirees the opportunity to receive increased pension benefits or benefits under an ESOP or other defined contribution retirement plan in exchange for or in lieu of certain employer-provided health benefits.

Table 10.4 shows some advantages and disadvantages of providing cash or other benefits in lieu of retiree health benefits.

TABLE 10.4 **Cash or Other Benefits**

Advantages	Disadvantages
☐ Avoids costs associated with future health care inflation.	☐ Cash-out value is difficult to estimate and may be very costly.
☐ May enable company to make use of surplus pension assets by increasing pension benefits.	☐ Company not guaranteed that retirees will use amounts to purchase health care.
☐ Tax-favored funding exists from the employer's perspective.	☐ Company will probably still need to make available group vehicle to have retirees buy coverage in a cost-effective manner.
	☐ Future legislation could affect technique both favorably and unfavorably.
	☐ Retiree generally taxed on cash or pension amounts used to purchase health care, whereas health benefit coverage provided by an employer is generally nontaxable.

Managed Care

As part of a cost containment strategy, many companies have already implemented "managed care" programs to better control utilization of health care services by their active and retired employees. However, many of these techniques may not achieve significant cost savings with respect to Medicare-eligible retirees (those over age 65), since Medicare includes managed care features. However, managed care may be appropriate for non-Medicare eligible retirees.

Alternative Delivery Systems

Retirees can be enrolled in various alternative delivery systems including:

- ☐ HMOs (health maintenance organizations);
- ☐ PPOs (preferred provider organizations);
- ☐ direct contracting with local providers; and
- ☐ centers of excellence.

When analyzing various alternative delivery systems as part of a cost containment strategy, important considerations include the following.

- Demographics and utilization patterns of the retiree group.
- Retiree reluctance to switch from traditional indemnity programs.
- Geographic location of HMOs and PPOs and geographic concentrations of retirees.
- PPO utilization controls, which directly impact company savings.
- Appropriateness of providing certain ancillary benefits, such as vision and dental care, to retirees.
- A company's ability to access and evaluate data from providers.

Utilization Review Programs
Utilization review services can be used with indemnity plans to reduce unnecessary use of health care services and thereby reduce costs. Among the more common techniques used with indemnity plans for retirees are hospital preadmission certification, concurrent review, second surgical opinions, and discharge planning. These techniques may be cost effective for retirees under age 65 who generally have more claims for hospitalization than do active employees. However, utilization review for retirees over age 65 may not be cost effective, since the Medicare program already includes certain utilization review features. In addition, some utilization review techniques shift costs away from Medicare and onto the company.

Large Case Management
Chronic illnesses account for a significant portion of medical expenditures because treatment is not provided in the most cost-effective location. Large case management identifies individuals with chronic conditions and then attempts to direct care to the most cost-effective setting, such as a skilled nursing facility or home, with home health services instead of remaining in the hospital.

Medicare Risk Contracts and Medicare Insured Groups
Several relatively recent developments in "managed care" involve the provision of prepaid Medicare services through private health plans or HMOs, and may provide companies with plan design opportunities. HMOs or competitive medical plans (CMPs) with Medicare Risk Contracts can receive a per capita payment for Medicare enrollees equal to 95 percent of the average cost of Medicare benefits in the community. The HMO must then cover Medicare Part A and Part B services.

Companies can coordinate their retiree health benefit programs with Medicare Risk Contracts by paying all or part of the premium for additional services not covered by Medicare. Company premiums could be reduced if there are savings under the Medicare contract. This arrangement can provide companies with additional strength in negotiating with HMOs for favorable premium rates.

Medicare Insured Groups or MIGs are plans operated by large employers or unions that combine Medicare and supplemental benefit plans into a single insurance plan. Proponents claim that MIGs can ensure continuity of care for retirees, eliminate multiple claims, and can give companies additional leverage in negotiating with providers. In MIGs, enrollees must be given a choice between indemnity (fee-for-service) and alternative delivery system arrangements. The MIG will be paid 95 percent of the average cost of Medicare benefits for the plan's retirees on an experience rated basis. If the MIG operates at a lower cost than the Medicare capitation payments, it may keep up to 5 percent of the excess; any additional savings must be used to provide additional benefits.

Constraints

The health care benefits environment is complex and rapidly changing, as the economic, regulatory, and business forces affecting plans continue to change. A company must address various factors, both internal (e.g., demographics, collective bargaining agreements, resources available for benefits) and external (e.g., legal issues, delivery of health care, cost trends) in making plan design decisions. Some of the key issues are discussed below.

Demographic and Claims Data

There is a critical link between plan design changes and analysis of the current and projected retiree population and health care claims costs. For example, a company considering dollar-denominated benefits must understand its retiree health claims data to select the appropriate dollar level of benefits. A company considering a PPO arrangement for retirees must determine whether enough retirees reside in the PPO's geographic area to make it a worthwhile option. Similarly, understanding costs by health care service sector may help a company to evaluate increased cost sharing, managed care, and case management techniques.

Even if no plan design changes are made, good quality data will help management better understand how their company is spending money on health care and the data that will be needed for effective cost management and funding strategies.

There are a number of actions that a company can take to improve its controls over data and plan administration. For example, an audit of a company's health care claims is an effective means of monitoring the way health plans are administered. A claims audit can achieve short-term objectives of improving basic controls, accuracy and efficiency of claims payment, and quality of data.

A complete claims audit normally covers several steps:

- define objectives and scope of audit;
- scrutinize computer and management functions—the most critical control areas;
- build a framework of the audit;
- examine sample claims; and
- analyze findings and recommendations.

Claims audits can achieve short-term benefits by recovering overpaid claims or other prior errors of the administrator. Future savings can be realized through identification and correction of procedural problems and by strengthening controls. Other savings may result from identification of utilization patterns. If no problems are identified, claims audits can reaffirm management's choice of administrator and other internal controls.

Employee Relations

A company's benefits philosophy will, of course, strongly influence its consideration of plan design options. A company that believes employees should have the freedom to choose among providers may wish to offer retirees several options, perhaps a plan that allows employees to choose among different types of benefits, with health care as one option. A company that believes retirees should be encouraged to be efficient health care consumers may wish to promote health awareness and increase cost sharing.

Companies also need to be aware of the needs and concerns of retirees and their union or nonunion representatives, as well as active employees who will be concerned about the security of their benefits upon retirement. Finally, a company must carefully review its collective bargaining agreements and consider future negotiations to determine its latitude in making plan design changes. Cost containment programs may have to be phased in according to priorities established by management in cooperation with employee groups.

Legal Issues

Employers have generally believed that they have great flexibility in setting eligibility requirements and controlling modification or termination of retiree health plans. While this may be true with respect to future benefits for active employees, recent court decisions indicate that the issue is much more complex. Beginning in 1983 with the decision in *UAW v. Yard-Man, Inc.,* followed shortly thereafter by *Eardman v. Bethlehem Steel, Inc.* and other cases, courts in several instances have found that retirees had contractual rights to welfare benefits, determined by the terms of plan documents and relevant collective bargaining agreements. Where union member retirees were involved, several courts concluded that retiree benefits continue beyond the expiration of the collective bargaining agreement. In most cases, absent clear, unambiguous statements reserving the right to modify or terminate benefits, there is an effective presumption that the benefits survive the agreement.

More recently, in the 1988 *Alpha Portland* cases, the U.S. Court of Appeals for the 8th Circuit concluded that the plan documents provided that their terms could be amended, modified or supplemented, and relevant bargaining agreements reflected an intent to limit the term of coverage. Therefore, retiree welfare benefits did not "vest," nor was the employer contractually obligated to provide such benefits to current retirees. Similarly, *Moore v. Metropolitan Life* in the U.S. Court of Appeals in the Second Circuit and, in the Sixth Circuit, *Musto v. American General,* both decided in 1988, upheld the employer's ability to modify or terminate retiree health benefits with respect to current retirees where the right to do so had been clearly reserved.

Observation: Perhaps, at least two lessons can be drawn from these cases. First, generally under current case law, the employer's legal commitment appears to be very much dependent on its verbal and written representations, and explicit reservation of the right to terminate or modify the plan is essential. Second, the legal theories supporting these decisions are still not fully settled.

This uncertain legal climate means that employers must plan carefully and consult legal counsel as they consider the future of their retiree health benefit programs. At a minimum, management will need to examine the benefits program for retirees by analyzing existing plan documents, summary plan descriptions, as well as procedures for exit interviews, retirement seminars, and all other relevant oral and written communications.

Nondiscrimination Rules for Welfare Plans (IRC Section 89)

The new nondiscrimination rules for welfare plans (Section 89 of the Internal Revenue Code) add another layer of complexity to the task of assessing an employer's current plans and options. These rules, which are generally effective for plan years beginning in 1989, require employers to undertake complex testing to determine whether their health (and group-term life insurance) plans discriminate in favor of highly compensated employees.

Under the §89 rules, health plans for "former employees" such as retirees and terminated disabled employees must be tested completely separately from active employees. When testing the former employee group, employees who terminated employment prior to January 1, 1989 (and have not been reemployed by the employer) may be disregarded in applying the nondiscrimination rules, unless benefits are increased or modified on a discriminatory basis (unless modified to comply with a federal law such as the Medicare Catastrophic Coverage Act).

Certain disparities in benefits or coverage are permissible under the nondiscrimination rules. For example, a health plan may be coordinated with Medicare as long as the method of coordination does not discriminate in favor of highly compensated employees. Under this rule, a retiree health plan apparently could provide one level of benefits for retirees under age 65 and a lower level of benefits for retirees age 65 and over who are enrolled in Medicare, as long as the manner of coordination did not discriminate in favor of highly compensated employees.

Observation: At this time, the application of the §89 nondiscrimination rules to retiree health plans is somewhat unclear. The law and its legislative history provide little guidance, and the §89 regulations issued by the Treasury Department in March 1989 did not address this area. Moreover, legislative and regulatory efforts to delay or modify §89 have intensified.

Despite the lack of guidance, it seems that the §89 rules will impact retiree health plans, and may make certain plan design options impractical for some employers. Some of the situations that may require special scrutiny follow.

- Failure to make health coverage available to at least 90 percent of the nonhighly compensated retirees.
- Differences in plan eligibility or benefits for groups of former employees, such as

    —executive only retiree plans;

    —plans that grade benefits with length of service;

    —union and nonunion plans; and

    —early retirement incentive programs.

- Post-1988 plan design changes modifying benefits for pre-1989 retirees.

Impact on Other Benefits

In making the transition to a new retiree health plan, a company must, of course, be sensitive to the different concerns of retirees, active employees nearing retirement, and younger active employees. Changes in the retiree health plan may affect the compensation or benefits program for active employees. In some cases, health plans for active employees may have to be modified to reflect the changes to the retiree health plan (e.g., establishing flexible benefit plans for both active and retired employees).

Plan modifications could have a profound effect on current retirees and employees nearing retirement who have depended on the retiree health care program in their financial planning for retirement.

Observation: Depending upon an employer's situation, it may be appropriate, therefore, to "grandfather" benefits for such individuals by, for example:

- *continuing to maintain the plan for current retirees;*

- *granting current retirees and those within, for example, three years of retirement, a minimum credit for service or reduced contributions under the new plan; or*

- *implementing changes gradually over a period of years.*

Long-Term Outlook

Companies will need to consider a number of long-term factors in designing a strategy to deal with retiree health benefits.

Medicare Erosion

In recent years, Medicare has raised premiums and deductibles, shifting more costs to employers and Medicare enrollees. In addition, Medicare has become secondary payer in certain instances, leaving employers primarily responsible for the health care costs of certain Medicare-eligible beneficiaries. In all likelihood, Medicare benefits will continue to erode, with more and more costs shifted to retirees and employers, and companies will need to continue to consider this trend as they look at various strategies.

The Changing Health Care Environment

The rapid and continuous changes in our health care environment affect plan design decisions and their implementation. Employers and their advisers must consider many factors, some quantifiable and some not, in assessing and implementing plan design options, including, for example:

- the effect of advances in technology and changing patterns of disease on costs, life expectancy, and standards of care;
- the tension between provider efforts to maximize reimbursement and payer efforts to hold down costs, such as Medicare DRGs;
- cost shifting from employers with discounted provider arrangements to those without discounted arrangements; and
- provision of benefits for the uninsured and underinsured.

Management should realistically evaluate the company's total compensation and benefits package needed to attract and retain the quality employees needed to remain competitive in the longer term.

Dedicated and realistic approaches that are applied to other key business planning issues are needed to establish an effective strategy for managing health care costs. It will clearly be a challenge for companies to provide health care programs that are responsive to retirees' and employees' needs, but at the same time are manageable, efficient, and cost effective.

11
Funding and Legislative Outlook

Currently most companies do not prefund retiree health benefits, generally because there are few tax incentives to do so. However, many companies are interested in advance funding their retiree health benefits to secure payment of those benefits, and to establish a plan asset under the ED for financial reporting purposes, thereby reducing the net recorded liability on the balance sheet. The expected return on plan assets would also be an offset (reduction) in computing annual expense under the ED.

The ED provides that, for financial reporting purposes, plan assets would have to be segregated and restricted (usually in a trust) to be used only for postretirement benefits. Assets that are not effectively restricted (so that they cannot be used by the employer for other purposes) are not plan assets for purposes of the ED, and could not offset reported liabilities. Accordingly, employers will generally want to evaluate whether a particular funding mechanism will be considered a plan asset, and will want to compare the financial returns and related attributes of each available funding option.

As a general matter, there is so much change and activity in the retiree health benefits area—proposed new accounting, changes in Medicare, congressional interest—that companies may want to remain flexible, and may be reluctant to make a substantial financial commitment to fund at this time.

This chapter briefly describes various funding options, their advantages and disadvantages, and discusses the legislative outlook for new funding proposals.

Funding Options

Section 401(h) Accounts

Retiree health benefits can be prefunded through a separate account in a qualified pension plan, known as a "Section 401(h) account." Section 401(h) accounts provide limited tax-favored opportunities for prefunding sickness, accident, hospitalization and medical expenses for retired employees, their spouses, and their dependents. A separate recordkeeping account must be maintained for those contributions used to fund retiree health benefits. All amounts in the §401(h) account must be used to provide health-related benefits for retirees, their spouses, and dependents. In addition, the employer may not receive a reversion of excess assets from the §401(h) account until all liabilities for retiree medical benefits are satisfied.

Tax-deductible employer contributions are made to a §401(h) account on an actuarial basis (including health care trend assumptions), and earnings in the account accumulate tax free. However, medical benefits must remain incidental to pension benefits under the pension plan. Under this rule, employer contributions to a §401(h) account are generally limited to 25 percent of the aggregate employer contributions to the plan since the beginning of the plan year of adoption of the §401(h) benefits. In the past, the Internal Revenue Service has taken the position that companies that cannot make pension contributions (because their pension plans have reached the full funding limit of 150 percent of current pension liabilities to employees and beneficiaries) are unable to make deductible contributions to §401(h) accounts. This limitation severely restricted the use of §401(h) accounts for many companies.

Recently, the IRS National Office appears to have shifted its position. In several private letter rulings and a General Counsel's Memorandum,[1] the IRS has permitted companies with pension plans at or near the full funding limit to make deductible §401(h) contributions based on the pension plan's "normal cost" under the projected unit credit method, rather than actual pension contributions. Reasonable assumptions must be used regarding the medical benefits, coverage, and funding medium. While IRS private letter rulings may only be relied upon by the companies to whom they were issued, this shift of position is viewed by many as a very promising development.

Table 11.1 summarizes some of the advantages and disadvantages of §401(h) accounts.

TABLE 11.1 §401(h) Accounts

Advantages	Disadvantages
☐ Employer contributions are tax deductible (within limits).	☐ Amounts restricted to use for health benefits.
☐ Earnings on plan assets generally not taxed.	☐ No direct transfer from pension plan or VEBA.
☐ Health care inflation can be considered.	☐ No guarantee of benefits by Pension Benefit Guaranty Corporation.
☐ Aggregate limits keyed to year of adoption of §401(h) account so that flexibility in contribution levels may be permitted.	☐ Separate recordkeeping account required.
☐ Most likely a plan asset under the ED, since amounts must be used to provide postretirement medical benefits (i.e., segregated and restricted).	☐ Separate subaccounts must be established for "key employees," and contributions to individual medical benefit accounts in a pension plan count as annual additions for purposes of Internal Revenue Code §415.
☐ Medical benefits excluded from income of retiree, spouse, and dependents.	☐ Historically limited usefulness for companies with fully funded pension plans, but IRS has apparent change in position.

VEBAs

Voluntary Employees' Beneficiary Associations (known as VEBAs or §501(c)(9) trusts) may be established to provide life, sickness, accident, or other welfare benefits, including retiree health benefits. Prior to the 1984 Deficit Reduction Act (DEFRA), VEBAs had tax advantages similar to pension trusts—employer contributions were tax deductible and trust earnings were not taxed.

However, DEFRA imposed significant limitations on the tax benefits and prefunding opportunities available to VEBAs (and other funded welfare benefit plans), some of which are discussed below.

In general, the Internal Revenue Code limits the deduction for contributions to a VEBA in a particular year to amounts reasonably and actuarially necessary to fund claims incurred during the year (i.e., current costs) and administrative expenses with respect to those claims. A VEBA may contain a reserve for postretirement medical benefits, funded on a level actuarial basis over the working lives of covered employees. However, this reserve is to be determined on the basis of current costs only (i.e., no health care inflation assumption is permitted), so that prefunding opportunities are limited. Moreover, benefits to be provided by the reserve may not discriminate in favor of highly compensated employees.

The IRS has issued virtually no guidance with respect to the actuarial methodology for funding retiree health benefits through a VEBA.[2] In particular, the IRS has not stated how much latitude companies have in the selection of:

- ☐ funding (attribution) method;
- ☐ amortization periods; or
- ☐ assumptions.

In addition, the IRS has not provided guidance on when it would consider a plan providing retiree health benefits to be a plan of deferred compensation and when it would be considered a welfare benefit plan. Accordingly, these issues should be carefully considered when evaluating any VEBA funding option.

In a VEBA that contains a reserve for postretirement medical benefits, investment income to the VEBA is generally taxable as unrelated business taxable income (UBTI). The VEBA trust would generally be taxed at trust rates. Accordingly, the ability to accumulate funds on a tax-free basis in a VEBA may be largely eliminated.

Under a special Internal Revenue Code provision (and pending issuance of IRS regulations on this provision), a fund maintained under a collective bargaining agreement is not subject to these deduction limits on funding. Moreover, investment income to such a fund is tax exempt. In addition, a collectively bargained plan is not subject to the requirement that the reserve must be nondiscriminatory. Therefore, funding through a VEBA may be an attractive option for retiree health benefits under a collective bargaining agreement.

For financial reporting purposes, it is possible under the ED that amounts in the VEBA may be considered plan assets, if they are maintained exclusively to pay retiree health benefits. The specific facts and circumstances relating to a VEBA will, of course, be crucial in determining whether the VEBA holdings would be considered plan assets. If these funds are not considered plan assets, the company's contributions to the VEBA could be considered to be assets of the sponsoring
company.

Tax-Exempt VEBA Investments
It should be noted that there are a number of investment strategies commonly associated with VEBAs, including various life insurance products and tax-exempt municipal bonds, that generally would not produce taxable income for the VEBA under current law. Many of these investments can require substantial initial cash

outlays and a long-term commitment. Therefore, projected cash flow requirements relating to the obligations funded by the VEBA should be carefully evaluated and appropriately linked to the projections of investment results and cash flows.

There are various tax and economic factors to consider when evaluating these investment options, including:

- Tax treatment of the various features of the investment product (e.g., surrender or withdrawal charges on insurance contracts).

- Risk of change in tax treatment of product (e.g., renewed legislative proposals—that have not in the past been successful—to curtail the tax-free "inside buildup" in cash surrender value in life insurance contracts).

- Whether insurance contracts comply with federal and state law requirements (e.g., is there an "insurable interest").

- Projected investment returns (e.g., when does tax-exempt return equal or exceed after-tax yield on taxable investments).

- ERISA fiduciary rules (e.g., prudence, diversification, prohibited transactions) that govern investment decisions of pension or welfare benefit fund fiduciaries (including a retiree health benefit fund).

Profit-Sharing Plans or Savings Accounts

A number of companies have expressed interest in establishing or amending profit-sharing plans to allow employees to leave a portion of their accounts in the plan to pay for health care during retirement. Under this "defined contribution" approach, a company could increase its tax-deductible contributions to the plan to include an amount for retiree health benefits, although overall limits on deductions to profit-sharing plans (i.e., generally 15 percent of payroll) would still apply. In addition, annual contributions on behalf of an individual to such a profit-sharing plan, together with annual contributions allocated on behalf of that individual to other profit-sharing, money purchase or stock bonus plans, are generally limited to the lesser of (a) $30,000 or (b) 25 percent of the individual's compensation for the year. Important issues to consider in evaluating this funding option include:

- Impact on tax-qualified status of profit-sharing plan by including retiree health benefit feature.

- Tax consequences to employees (retirees) of employer contributions intended to provide retiree health benefits and of amounts used to pay for retiree health benefits.
- Restrictions on amounts for retiree health benefits that would impact treatment of related profit-sharing plan assets as a plan asset under the ED.
- Possible IRS ruling clarifying the tax results relating to such an arrangement.

Because of these and other unresolved issues, many employers are waiting for regulatory guidance and perhaps even legislative guidance before establishing or amending profit-sharing plans to provide retiree health benefits.

Corporate-Owned Life Insurance

Some companies have purchased corporate-owned life insurance (COLI) policies on the lives of employees or retirees to provide future cash flows for retiree health benefits. These life insurance products are often leveraged, with partially or fully tax-deductible policy loans used by the corporate owner to pay non-tax-deductible premiums. Under current law, the cash value of the policy (inside buildup) accumulates tax free. The company intends to hold these policies until the death of the insured employee, at which time the proceeds are used to pay retiree health benefits.

There are many factors to consider when evaluating the use of COLI as an investment to provide future cash flows for retiree health benefits, including the following:

- A $50,000 limit on the amount of policy loans for each insured individual limits the deductibility of interest payments and the leveraging benefits of COLI, and also requires the purchase of a large number of insurance policies.
- As with some other funding alternatives, COLI would be a long-term commitment with substantial initial outlay.
- Possible tax law changes that may limit the tax advantages of this type of insurance investment.
- COLI would not be considered a plan asset under the ED, unless it is segregated and restricted from the employer's general assets only to pay benefits under the plan.

Group Health Insurance

In certain situations, such as plan terminations and acquisitions, a company may be able to purchase group health insurance with a long-term rate guarantee that allows for a transfer of liability to the insurer for benefits covered in the insurance contract. In effect, such a contract is somewhat like a single premium annuity. The contract could cover specified benefits, and perhaps could even anticipate changes in coverage. To assume this risk, the insurer would require the obligation to be very carefully measured, and might require the company to remain liable for benefits created by certain changes, such as decreased Medicare payments. For financial reporting purposes, under the ED this type of arrangement probably would not be treated as a settlement unless all significant risk is transferred to the insurer. Moreover, this type of insurance is generally not available, and may be prohibitively priced due to the insurer's perceived risk.

Legislative Outlook

There have been several recent proposals to provide tax incentives for funding retiree health benefits. Most notable are the various proposals that would permit companies to transfer surplus pension assets to fund retiree health benefits, and the proposal of Congressman Chandler (R-WA) to expand §401(h) accounts and permit asset transfers to fund retiree health benefits.

The transfer of surplus pension assets would allow some companies to satisfy a portion of their retiree health obligations while maintaining a strong funding position for their pension benefits. Under a proposal of the Coalition for Retirement Income Security (CRIS—a group of over a dozen large companies), companies could voluntarily dedicate surplus pension assets to fund retiree health benefits, but they would not have to pay income or excise taxes on the transfer (which would be the case if the employer directly recovered surplus pension assets in a reversion). The transfer proposed by CRIS would not force vesting or annuitization of active or retiree pension liabilities as would complete termination of the pension plan to recover the surplus.

According to CRIS, the federal government would realize increased revenues of $6.5 to $7 billion over five fiscal years, as companies paid health benefits out of trust assets and ceased taking current tax deductions for retiree health benefit expenditures.

The transfer proposal is not an ongoing funding mechanism, but a limited opportunity for companies to efficiently satisfy a large portion of their retiree health obligations. Benefit security for that portion of the obligation would be achieved immediately, rather than over a longer time period as under other funding mechanisms. The transfer of surplus assets to fund retiree health obligations would also diminish the availability of those assets for use in leveraged buyouts, or for other purposes which many argue are not in the best interests of plan participants.

The proposals currently under discussion involve the voluntary dedication of surplus pension assets to fund retiree health obligations. Under one proposal, only transfers to fund retiree health or long-term care, or employee stock ownership plans (ESOPs) would be permitted—all other plan terminations with reversions of surplus pension assets would be subject to a 100 percent excise tax. Another proposal would raise the current 150 percent full funding limit to 200 percent, and would permit tax-free reversions where at least 50 percent of the reversion amount is used to fund retiree health benefits.

Current proposals for ongoing funding are primarily based on expansion of current funding mechanisms. For example, Congressman Chandler's bill creates additional opportunities for prefunding retiree health and long-term care benefits through §401(h) accounts. However, many are concerned about ERISA-like minimum participation and vesting standards that might apply to the benefits funded.

Any legislative efforts to provide tax incentives for funding retiree health benefits will confront several major impediments.

- Congress and the administration are likely to be preoccupied with the federal budget deficit. Because of concerns over the fiscal effect of additional tax incentives, such as those for funding retiree health benefits, these proposals are unlikely to gain support without offsetting revenue enhancements. Prefunding proposals generate revenue loss by accelerating deductibility of employer contributions and permitting tax-free earnings of funds set aside for this purpose.

- Congress is likely to focus on broader health care issues—such as mandated employer-provided health benefits, problems of the uninsured, and long-term care—rather than legislation specifically dealing with funding for employer-provided retiree health benefits.

- Congress may be more interested in adjustments to the Medicare Catastrophic Coverage Act or efforts to provide other benefits through Medicare (e.g., long-term care).

Conclusion

Although some have stated that the FASB Exposure Draft has provided an impetus for companies to explore funding vehicles, many argue that it is unlikely that any new laws allowing tax-favored funding of retiree health benefits will be enacted in the near future. Therefore, companies may wish to consider flexible interim solutions and evaluate the following strategies to determine the most advantageous way to discharge future obligations.

- Assess funding alternatives allowed under current law.
- Monitor the progress of proposed legislation.
- Analyze potential new funding vehicles.
- Consider making company views known to Congress regarding desired tax incentives for advance funding.

Notes

1. I.R.S. General Counsel's Memorandum 39785, March 24, 1989.
2. The IRS has informally indicated that terminal funding (i.e., fund completely at retirement) for retiree health benefits would be impermissible.

12
Profiles of the Field Test Companies

The impact of applying the ED to a specific company depends on several factors, including the nature of the benefits provided, the demographic characteristics of the plan population, and the actuarial assumptions used to measure obligations and expense. Therefore, individual profiles were prepared for a representative sample of companies participating in the Field Test to give readers a sense of some of the key factors that may affect the measurement of retiree health benefits. The underlying data for each profile was developed from the actuarial valuation reports that were completed for each Field Test company. The sample companies were selected and the underlying data summarized so as to preserve the anonymity of the participating companies.

Nearly all of the Field Test companies are mature or highly mature with plans that have been in existence for many years. Accordingly, the ED's impact on the financial statements of the Field Test companies may not be indicative of the financial statement effect on less mature companies. In addition, since the impact is dependent on the specific benefits offered by the company as well as on its demographic make-up, companies should be cautious in extrapolating the Field Test results to their circumstances.

To assess how the ED would affect a specific company, the company would need to apply the ED to its own plan, demographics, and current health care claims experience.

Organization of Company Profiles

As discussed in chapter 4, the Field Test companies have defined the term "plan" differently. For purposes of the profiles presented in this chapter, information on more than one plan was generally combined. In addition, in completing the company profile, if any portion of a company's retiree health program satisfied a question, the question was answered "yes." For example, in the plan characteristics section, the question is posed: "Are any direct contributions required?" If any retirees were required to contribute any amount, a "yes" was included.

The profiles of the Field Test companies have been organized based on the relationship of retirees (excluding dependents) to active employees (including actives fully eligible), as follows:

- Highly Mature—Company 1 through 4—less than two active employees for every retiree.
- Mature—Company 5 through 10—two to six active employees for every retiree.
- Immature—Company 11 through 12—more than six active employees for every retiree.

Within each individual company profile, the following data has been presented:

Plan characteristics. Includes basic information on overall provisions of the retiree health plans offered. This section also provides the company's Medicare integration approach (see chapter 10 for discussion of alternative approaches).

1988 pay-as-you-go costs per capita. Includes 1988 estimated pay-as-you-go costs per capita (based on retirees and dependents combined)[1], as follows:

- high—$2,500 or greater;
- medium—between $1,500 and $2,500; and
- low—below $1,500.

Transition periods. Includes the average remaining service period (ARSP) under the ED based on the date of full eligibility and the date of expected retirement (excluding the impact of the optional 15-year period).

Participants receiving benefits. Includes demographic data on plan participants (retirees and dependents) currently receiving benefits.[1]

Actuarial assumptions. Includes the weighted average health care cost trend and discount rate assumptions used in analyzing the ED's impact.

Obligations at date of adoption. Includes the accumulated postretirement benefit obligation (APBO) at date of adoption expressed as a multiple of estimated pay-as-you-go costs for the year as follows:

- ☐ high—greater than 32 times;
- ☐ medium—16 to 32 times; and
- ☐ low—less than 16 times.

Also included is the percentage breakdown of the components of the expected postretirement benefit obligation (EPBO) at date of adoption.

Expense. Includes expense under the ED in the year of adoption expressed as a multiple of estimated pay-as-you-go costs for the year and a percentage breakdown of expense in the year of adoption into its components (service cost, interest cost, and amortization of the transition obligation).

Note

1. It should be noted that for a number of Field Test companies, only dependents with health care claims were included, thus understating actual dependents covered under the plan. In these instances adjustments were made to the valuation methodology to appropriately reflect the dependents' obligation. In addition, in some instances surviving spouses could not be differentiated from retirees.

Company 1

Plan Characteristics

Coverage other than medical	None
Is lifetime coverage provided for:	
Retiree?	Yes
Spouse?	Yes
Are there any lifetime maximums?	Yes
Are any direct contributions currently required for:	
Retiree?	Yes
Spouse?	Yes
Does company pay any portion of Part B premium?	No
Medicare integration method	Carve-out

1988 Pay-As-You-Go Costs per Capita   Low

Transition Periods

ARSP (all plans combined):	
to eligibility date	13.6 years
to expected retirement	18.2 years

Plan Participants

Ratio of active employees to retirees	Highly Mature

Participants Receiving Benefits

Retirees	54.5%
Dependents	45.5%

Actuarial Assumptions

Weighted average health care cost trend:	
Best estimate	7.6%
Discount rate based on ED	10.0%

Obligations at Date of Adoption

APBO as multiple of pay-as-you-go costs	Medium

Profiles of the Field Test Companies

FIGURE 12.1 Components of EPBO

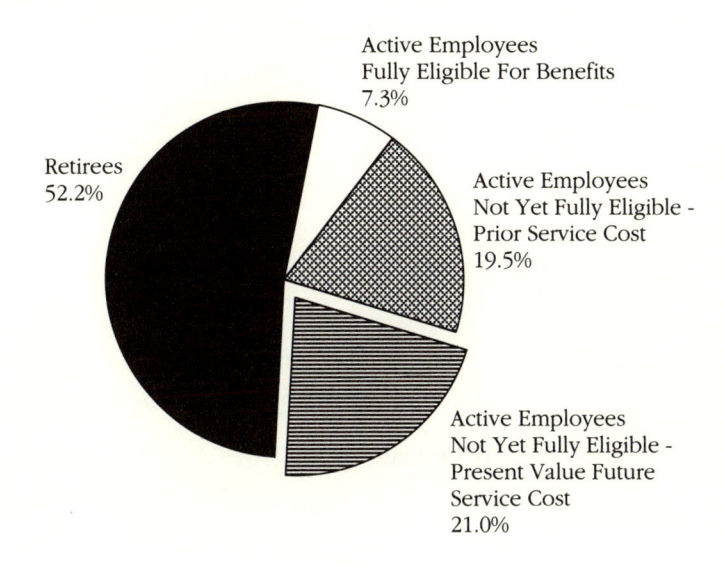

- Retirees 52.2%
- Active Employees Fully Eligible For Benefits 7.3%
- Active Employees Not Yet Fully Eligible - Prior Service Cost 19.5%
- Active Employees Not Yet Fully Eligible - Present Value Future Service Cost 21.0%

Expense under ED in Year of Adoption

Multiple of accrued expense to pay-as-you-go costs	3 times
Components of expense:	
Service cost	14.9%
Interest cost	54.5
Transition amortization	30.6
	100.0%

Company 2

Plan Characteristics

Coverage other than medical	None
Is lifetime coverage provided for:	
Retiree?	Yes
Spouse?	Yes
Are there any lifetime maximums?	Yes
Are any direct contributions currently required for:	
Retiree?	No
Spouse?	Yes
Does company pay any portion of Part B premium?	No
Medicare integration method	Carve-out

1988 Pay-As-You-Go Costs per Capita — Medium

Transition Periods

ARSP (all plans combined):
- to eligibility date — 10.9 years
- to expected retirement — 17.1 years

Plan Participants

Ratio of active employees to retirees — Highly Mature

Participants Receiving Benefits

Retirees	59.5%
Dependents	40.5%

Actuarial Assumptions

Weighted average health care cost trend:
- Best estimate — 7.9%
- Discount rate based on ED — 9.0%

Obligations at Date of Adoption

APBO as multiple of pay-as-you-go costs — Medium

FIGURE 12.2 **Components of EPBO**

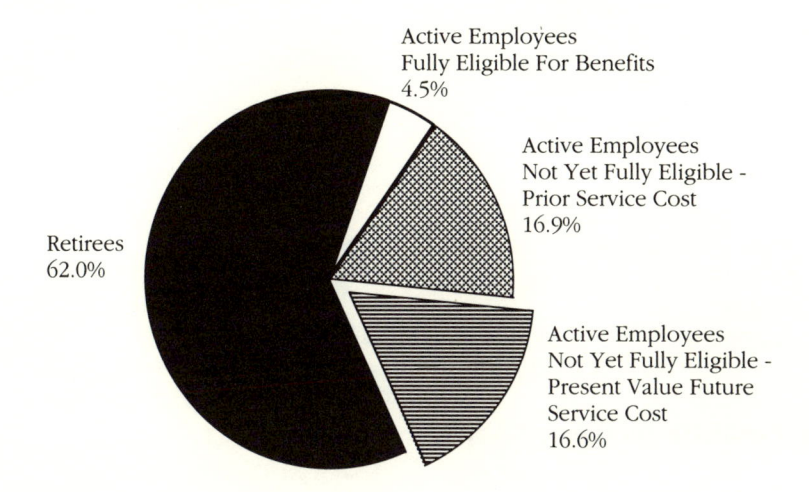

- Retirees 62.0%
- Active Employees Fully Eligible For Benefits 4.5%
- Active Employees Not Yet Fully Eligible - Prior Service Cost 16.9%
- Active Employees Not Yet Fully Eligible - Present Value Future Service Cost 16.6%

Expense under ED in Year of Adoption

Multiple of accrued expense to pay-as-you-go costs	3 times
Components of expense:	
Service cost	15.4%
Interest cost	50.8
Transition amortization	33.8
	100.0%

Company 3

Plan Characteristics

Coverage other than medical	Drugs
Is lifetime coverage provided for:	
Retiree?	Yes
Spouse?	Yes
Are there any lifetime maximums?	Yes
Are any direct contributions currently required for:	
Retiree?	Yes
Spouse?	Yes
Does company pay any portion of Part B premium?	No
Medicare integration method	Exclusion

1988 Pay-As-You-Go Costs per Capita — Low

Transition Periods

ARSP (all plans combined):	
to eligibility date	12.6 years
to expected retirement	14.7 years

Plan Participants

Ratio of active employees to retirees	Highly Mature

Participants Receiving Benefits

Retirees	57.4%
Dependents	42.6%

Actuarial Assumptions

Weighted average health care cost trend:	
Best estimate	7.9%
Discount rate based on ED	9.0%

Obligations at Date of Adoption

APBO as multiple of pay-as-you-go costs	Medium

FIGURE 12.3 **Components of EPBO**

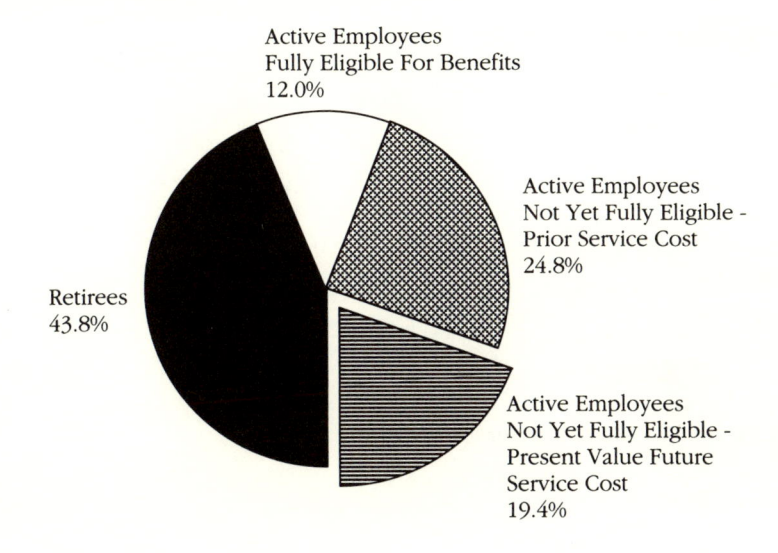

- Active Employees Fully Eligible For Benefits 12.0%
- Active Employees Not Yet Fully Eligible - Prior Service Cost 24.8%
- Active Employees Not Yet Fully Eligible - Present Value Future Service Cost 19.4%
- Retirees 43.8%

Expense under ED in Year of Adoption

Multiple of accrued expense to pay-as-you-go costs	4 times
Components of expense:	
Service cost	12.9%
Interest cost	49.6
Transition amortization	37.5
	100.0%

Company 4

Plan Characteristics

Coverage other than medical	Drugs
Is lifetime coverage provided for:	
Retiree?	Yes
Spouse?	Yes
Are there any lifetime maximums?	Yes
Are any direct contributions currently required for:	
Retiree?	No
Spouse?	No
Does company pay any portion of Part B premium?	Yes
Medicare integration method	Coordination

1988 Pay-As-You-Go Costs per Capita   Medium

Transition Periods

ARSP (all plans combined):	
to eligibility date	11.1 years
to expected retirement	13.8 years

Plan Participants

Ratio of active employees to retirees   Highly Mature

Participants Receiving Benefits

Retirees	49.2%
Dependents	50.8%

Actuarial Assumptions

Weighted average health care cost trend:	
Best estimate	6.9%
Discount rate based on ED	8.5%

Obligations at Date of Adoption

APBO as multiple of pay-as-you-go costs   Medium

FIGURE 12.4 **Components of EPBO**

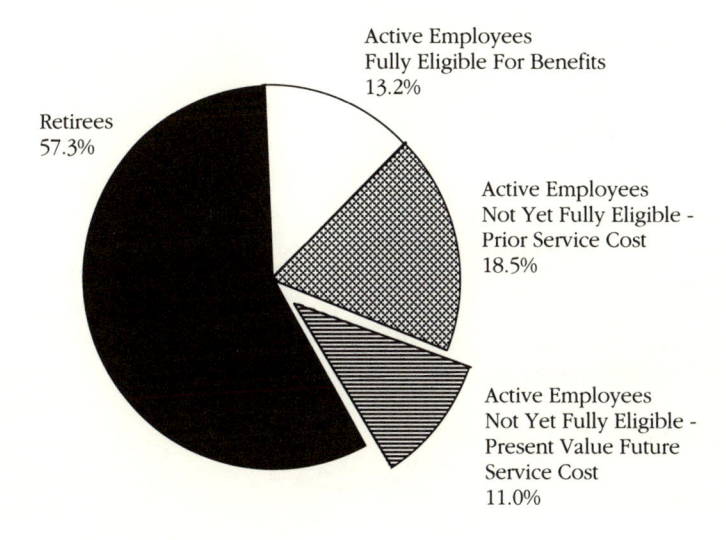

- Retirees 57.3%
- Active Employees Fully Eligible For Benefits 13.2%
- Active Employees Not Yet Fully Eligible - Prior Service Cost 18.5%
- Active Employees Not Yet Fully Eligible - Present Value Future Service Cost 11.0%

Expense under ED in Year of Adoption

Multiple of accrued expense to pay-as-you-go costs	3 times
Components of expense:	
Service cost	8.4%
Interest cost	50.7
Transition amortization	40.9
	100.0%

Company 5

Plan Characteristics

Coverage other than medical	None
Is lifetime coverage provided for:	
Retiree?	Yes
Spouse?	Yes
Are there any lifetime maximums?	Yes
Are any direct contributions currently required for:	
Retiree?	No
Spouse?	Yes
Does company pay any portion of Part B premium?	No
Medicare integration method	Exclusion

1988 Pay-As-You-Go Costs per Capita   Low

Transition Periods

ARSP (all plans combined):	
to eligibility date	15.9 years
to expected retirement	20.1 years

Plan Participants

Ratio of active employees to retirees	Mature

Participants Receiving Benefits

Retirees	55.9%
Dependents	44.1%

Actuarial Assumptions

Weighted average health care cost trend:	
Best estimate	8.9%
Discount rate based on ED	9.0%

Obligations at Date of Adoption

APBO as multiple of pay-as-you-go costs	High

FIGURE 12.5 Components of EPBO

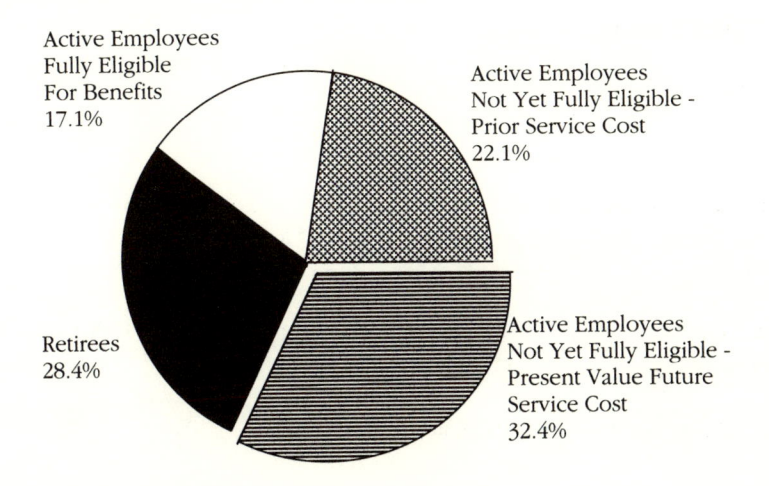

- Active Employees Fully Eligible For Benefits: 17.1%
- Active Employees Not Yet Fully Eligible - Prior Service Cost: 22.1%
- Active Employees Not Yet Fully Eligible - Present Value Future Service Cost: 32.4%
- Retirees: 28.4%

Expense under ED in Year of Adoption

Multiple of accrued expense to pay-as-you-go costs	8 times
Components of expense:	
Service cost	24.9%
Interest cost	48.2
Transition amortization	26.9
	100.0%

Company 6

Plan Characteristics

Coverage other than medical	Drugs, Dental
Is lifetime coverage provided for:	
Retiree?	Yes
Spouse?	No
Are there any lifetime maximums?	Yes
Are any direct contributions currently required for:	
Retiree?	Yes
Spouse?	Yes
Does company pay any portion of Part B premium?	No
Medicare integration method	Carve-out

1988 Pay-As-You-Go Costs per Capita   Low

Transition Periods

ARSP (all plans combined):	
to eligibility date	14.3 years
to expected retirement	19.8 years

Plan Participants

Ratio of active employees to retirees   Mature

Participants Receiving Benefits

Retirees	69.0%
Dependents	31.0%

Actuarial Assumptions

Weighted average health care cost trend:	
Best estimate	7.9%
Discount rate based on ED	9.25%

Obligations at Date of Adoption

APBO as multiple of pay-as-you-go costs   Medium

FIGURE 12.6 **Components of EPBO**

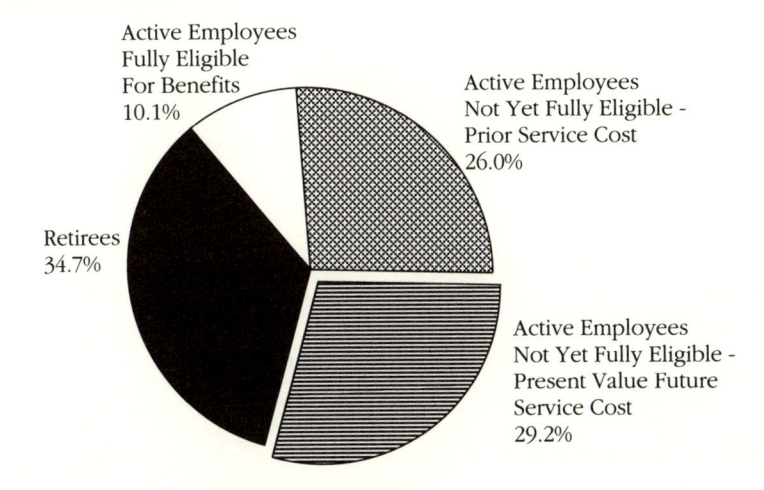

- Active Employees Fully Eligible For Benefits 10.1%
- Active Employees Not Yet Fully Eligible - Prior Service Cost 26.0%
- Retirees 34.7%
- Active Employees Not Yet Fully Eligible - Present Value Future Service Cost 29.2%

Expense under ED in Year of Adoption

Multiple of accrued expense to pay-as-you-go costs	5 times
Components of expense:	
Service cost	22.7%
Interest cost	49.7
Transition amortization	27.6
	100.0%

Company 7

Plan Characteristics

Coverage other than medical	Drugs, Dental
Is lifetime coverage provided for:	
Retiree?	Yes
Spouse?	No
Are there any lifetime maximums?	Yes
Are any direct contributions currently required for:	
Retiree?	Yes
Spouse?	Yes
Does company pay any portion of Part B premium?	Yes
Medicare integration method	Carve-out

1988 Pay-As-You-Go Costs per Capita — High

Transition Periods

ARSP (all plans combined):	
to eligibility date	10.4 years
to expected retirement	20.4 years

Plan Participants

Ratio of active employees to retirees	Mature

Participants Receiving Benefits

Retirees	56.3%
Dependents	43.7%

Actuarial Assumptions

Weighted average health care cost trend:	
Best estimate	8.0%
Discount rate based on ED	9.0%

Obligations at Date of Adoption

APBO as multiple of pay-as-you-go costs	Medium

FIGURE 12.7 **Components of EPBO**

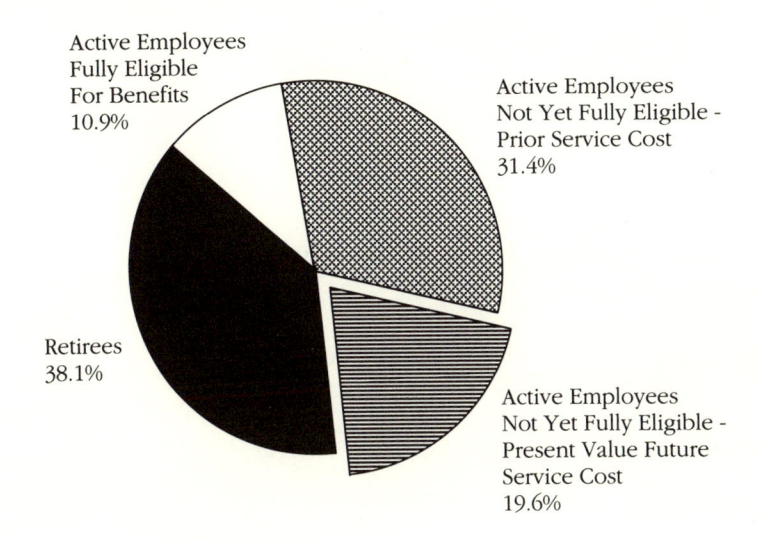

- Active Employees Fully Eligible For Benefits 10.9%
- Active Employees Not Yet Fully Eligible - Prior Service Cost 31.4%
- Active Employees Not Yet Fully Eligible - Present Value Future Service Cost 19.6%
- Retirees 38.1%

Expense under ED in Year of Adoption

Multiple of accrued expense to pay-as-you-go costs	4 times
Components of expense:	
Service cost	16.5%
Interest cost	53.7
Transition amortization	29.8
	100.0%

Company 8

Plan Characteristics

Coverage other than medical	None
Is lifetime coverage provided for:	
Retiree?	Yes
Spouse?	Yes
Are there any lifetime maximums?	Yes
Are any direct contributions currently required for:	
Retiree?	Yes
Spouse?	Yes
Does company pay any portion of Part B premium?	No
Medicare integration method	Carve-out

1988 Pay-As-You-Go Costs per Capita — Low

Transition Periods

ARSP (all plans combined):	
to eligibility date	13.7 years
to expected retirement	18.9 years

Plan Participants

Ratio of active employees to retirees	Mature

Participants Receiving Benefits

Retirees	68.4%
Dependents	31.6%

Actuarial Assumptions

Weighted average health care cost trend:	
Best estimate	8.2%
Discount rate based on ED	9.0%

Obligations at Date of Adoption

APBO as multiple of pay-as-you-go costs	Medium

FIGURE 12.8 **Components of EPBO**

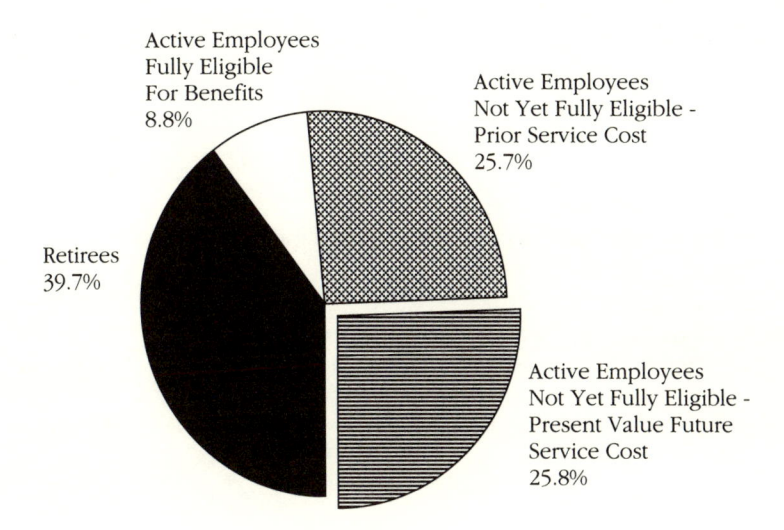

- Active Employees Fully Eligible For Benefits 8.8%
- Active Employees Not Yet Fully Eligible - Prior Service Cost 25.7%
- Retirees 39.7%
- Active Employees Not Yet Fully Eligible - Present Value Future Service Cost 25.8%

Expense under ED in Year of Adoption

Multiple of accrued expense to pay-as-you-go costs	5 times
Components of expense:	
Service cost	21.0%
Interest cost	49.4
Transition amortization	29.6
	100.0%

Company 9

Plan Characteristics

Coverage other than medical	Drugs, Dental
Is lifetime coverage provided for:	
Retiree?	Yes
Spouse?	No
Are there any lifetime maximums?	Yes
Are any direct contributions currently required for:	
Retiree?	Yes
Spouse?	Yes
Does company pay any portion of Part B premium?	No
Medicare integration method	Exclusion

1988 Pay-As-You-Go Costs per Capita   Medium

Transition Periods

ARSP (all plans combined):	
to eligibility date	13.0 years
to expected retirement	16.5 years

Plan Participants

Ratio of active employees to retirees   Mature

Participants Receiving Benefits

Retirees	59.2%
Dependents	40.8%

Actuarial Assumptions

Weighted average health care cost trend:	
Best estimate	6.3%
Discount rate based on ED	9.25%

Obligations at Date of Adoption

APBO as multiple of pay-as-you-go costs   Medium

FIGURE 12.9 **Components of EPBO**

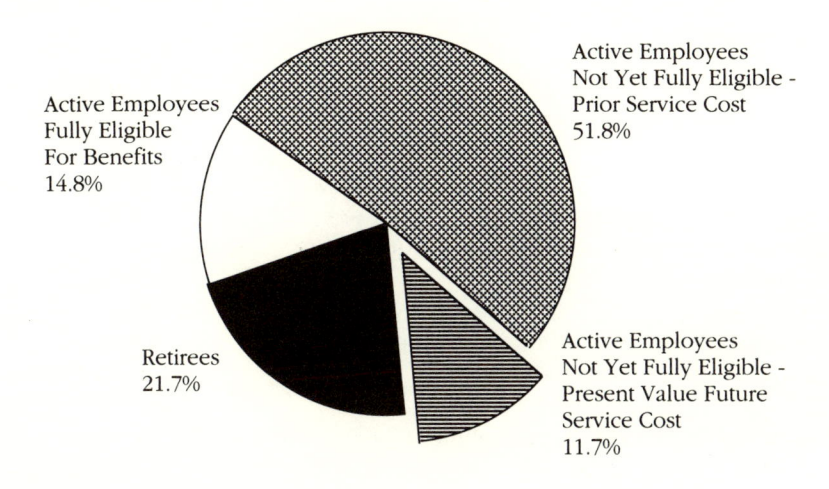

- Active Employees Fully Eligible For Benefits 14.8%
- Active Employees Not Yet Fully Eligible - Prior Service Cost 51.8%
- Retirees 21.7%
- Active Employees Not Yet Fully Eligible - Present Value Future Service Cost 11.7%

Expense under ED in Year of Adoption

Multiple of accrued expense to pay-as-you-go costs	4 times
Components of expense:	
Service cost	13.6%
Interest cost	51.8
Transition amortization	34.6
	100.0%

Company 10

Plan Characteristics

Coverage other than medical	Drugs
Is lifetime coverage provided for:	
Retiree?	Yes
Spouse?	No
Are there any lifetime maximums?	Yes
Are any direct contributions currently required for:	
Retiree?	No
Spouse?	No
Does company pay any portion of Part B premium?	No
Medicare integration method	Coordination

1988 Pay-As-You-Go Costs per Capita   Medium

Transition Periods

ARSP (all plans combined):	
to eligibility date	12.4 years
to expected retirement	19.7 years

Plan Participants

Ratio of active employees to retirees   Mature

Participants Receiving Benefits

Retirees	56.9%
Dependents	43.1%

Actuarial Assumptions

Weighted average health care cost trend:	
Best estimate	8.1%
Discount rate based on ED	8.75%

Obligations at Date of Adoption

APBO as multiple of pay-as-you-go costs   High

FIGURE 12.10 **Components of EPBO**

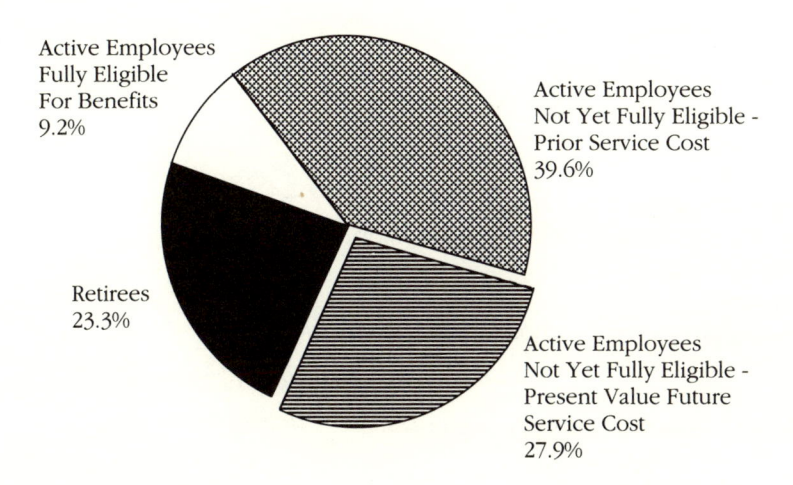

- Active Employees Fully Eligible For Benefits 9.2%
- Active Employees Not Yet Fully Eligible - Prior Service Cost 39.6%
- Retirees 23.3%
- Active Employees Not Yet Fully Eligible - Present Value Future Service Cost 27.9%

Expense under ED in Year of Adoption

Multiple of accrued expense to pay-as-you-go costs	7 times
Components of expense:	
Service cost	22.7%
Interest cost	48.7
Transition amortization	28.6
	100.0%

Company 11

Plan Characteristics

Coverage other than medical	Drugs
Is lifetime coverage provided for:	
Retiree?	Yes
Spouse?	Yes
Are there any lifetime maximums?	No
Are any direct contributions currently required for:	
Retiree?	Yes
Spouse?	Yes
Does company pay any portion of Part B premium?	No
Medicare integration method	Exclusion

1988 Pay-As-You-Go Costs per Capita — Low

Transition Periods

ARSP (all plans combined):	
to eligibility date	14.9 years
to expected retirement	20.2 years

Plan Participants

Ratio of active employees to retirees	Immature

Participants Receiving Benefits

Retirees	76.6%
Dependents	23.4%

Actuarial Assumptions

Weighted average health care cost trend:	
Best estimate	8.3%
Discount rate based on ED	7.5%

Obligations at Date of Adoption

APBO as multiple of pay-as-you-go costs	Medium

FIGURE 12.11 **Components of EPBO**

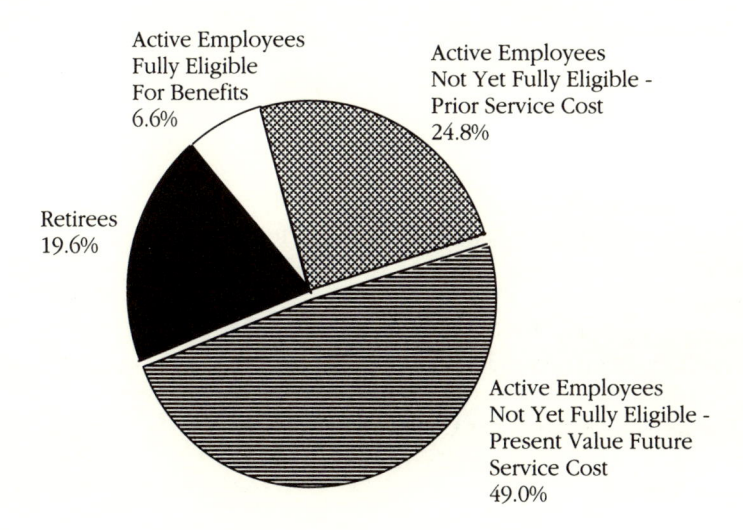

- Active Employees Fully Eligible For Benefits 6.6%
- Active Employees Not Yet Fully Eligible - Prior Service Cost 24.8%
- Retirees 19.6%
- Active Employees Not Yet Fully Eligible - Present Value Future Service Cost 49.0%

Expense under ED in Year of Adoption

Multiple of accrued expense to pay-as-you-go costs	6 times
Components of expense:	
Service cost	39.8%
Interest cost	36.0
Transition amortization	24.2
	100.0%

Company 12

Plan Characteristics

Coverage other than medical	Dental, Drugs
Is lifetime coverage provided for:	
Retiree?	Yes
Spouse?	Yes
Are there any lifetime maximums?	Yes
Are any direct contributions currently required for:	
Retiree?	No
Spouse?	No
Does company pay any portion of Part B premium?	No
Medicare integration method	Carve-out

1988 Pay-As-You-Go Costs per Capita   High

Transition Periods

ARSP (all plans combined):	
to eligibility date	12.0 years
to expected retirement	19.4 years

Plan Participants

Ratio of active employees to retirees   Immature

Participants Receiving Benefits

Retirees	49.0%
Dependents	51.0%

Actuarial Assumptions

Weighted average health care cost trend:	
Best estimate	8.1%
Discount rate based on ED	8.75%

Obligations at Date of Adoption

APBO as multiple of pay-as-you-go costs   High

FIGURE 12.12 **Components of EPBO**

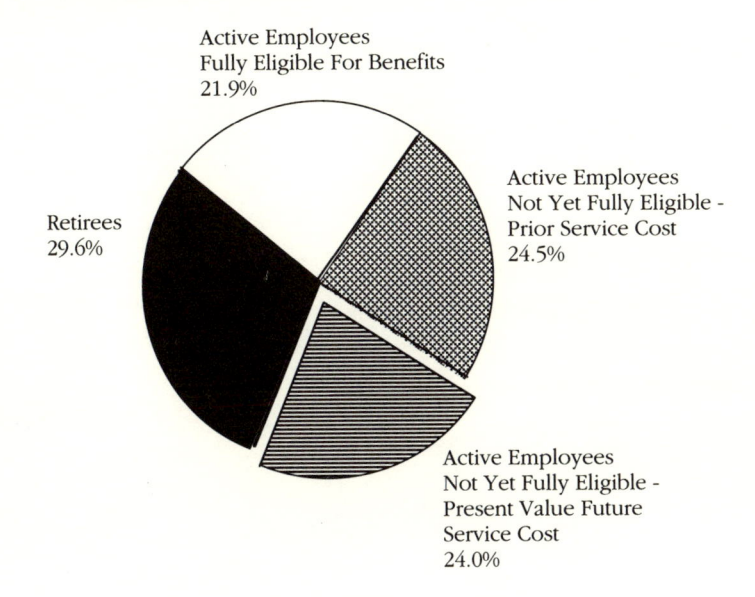

- Active Employees Fully Eligible For Benefits 21.9%
- Active Employees Not Yet Fully Eligible - Prior Service Cost 24.5%
- Active Employees Not Yet Fully Eligible - Present Value Future Service Cost 24.0%
- Retirees 29.6%

Expense under ED in Year of Adoption

Multiple of accrued expense to pay-as-you-go costs	7 times
Components of expense:	
Service cost	25.9%
Interest cost	42.0
Transition amortization	32.1
	100.0%